GP ST: Stage 2
Practice Questions

2009 edition

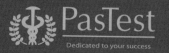

PasTest
Dedicated to your success

FOR SALE
£ 1.50

GP ST: Stage 2
Practice Questions

2009 edition

Edited by Sean Coughlin,
MBChB FRCGP MMedSc

General Practitioner

Lancashire

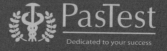

PasTest
Dedicated to your success

© 2008 PASTEST LTD
Egerton Court
Parkgate Estate
Knutsford
Cheshire
WA16 8DX

Telephone: 01565 752000

First Published 2007
Second Edition published 2008

ISBN: 1905 635 486

978 1905 635 481

A catalogue record for this book is available from the British Library.

The information contained within this book was obtained by the author from reliable sources. However, while every effort has been made to ensure its accuracy, no responsibility for loss, damage or injury occasioned to any person acting or refraining from action as a result of information contained herein can be accepted by the publishers or author.

PasTest Revision Books and Intensive Courses

PasTest has been established in the field of postgraduate medical education since 1972, providing revision books and intensive study courses for doctors preparing for their professional examinations.

Books and courses are available for the following specialties:
MRCGP, MRCP Parts 1 and 2, MRCPCH Parts 1 and 2, MRCPsych, MRCS, MRCOG Parts 1 and 2, DRCOG, DCH, FRCA, PLAB Parts 1 and 2.

For further details contact:

PasTest, Freepost, Knutsford, Cheshire WA16 7BR

Tel: 01565 752000 Fax: 01565 650264

www.pastest.co.uk enquiries@pastest.co.uk

Text prepared by Carnegie Book Production, Lancaster

Printed and bound by Page Bros, Norwich, UK

ajbdeane@doctors.org.uk

CONTENTS

CONTRIBUTORS

Paul Anderson, BSc (Hons), MB ChB (Hons), FRCS(Urol)
Consultant Urological Surgeon
Dudley

Angela Bennett, MB BChir
GP Registrar
York Street Medical Practice
Cambridge

Stephanie Coughlin MB BChir MA
Foundation Year 2
Emergency Department
Bedford Hospital
Bedford

Julia Dancy, MB ChB, MRCP (UK), DCH, DTM&H
GP Registrar
Croydon VTS
London Deanery

Arwa Eskander, MB ChB (Sheffield)
Foundation Year 2 Respiratory Medicine
University Hospital of North Staffordshire

Brandon John, MB ChB (Sheffield)
Foundation Year 2 Paediatrics
Stafford General Hospital
Stafford

Stephanie-Jayne Jones, BClin Sci, MB ChB, MRCP, MRCGP,
DipPharmMed
Sessional General Practitioner/Drug Safety Physician
Cheshire

Priya Joshi, MB ChB, DRCOG, MRCGP
Sessional General Practitioner
Cambridge

Louise Newson, BSc(Hons), MB ChB (Hons), MRCP MRCGP
General Practitioner
Solihull
West Midlands

Laura Weidner, MB ChB (UK)
Foundation Year 2 Doctor
Accident and Emergency
Walsall Hospitals NHS Trust
Walsall

INTRODUCTION

There is a nationally agreed and quality assured process of appointment to general practitioner (GP) specialty training, coordinated by the National Recruitment Office. Full details of the process can be found on the Office's website (www.gprecruitment.org.uk).

Currently, there are four stages in the process:

- Stage 1 (long-list) consists of filling an application form, providing personal and professional details. If a candidate's details meet the essential eligibility criteria, the application is accepted.

- Stage 2 (short-list) is an assessment conducted under exam conditions. The rest of this book is about this stage, and provides advice and material to help candidates prepare for and successfully negotiate the assessment.

- Stage 3 (selection) consists of an assessment at a selection centre. An invitation to attend will be sent to those candidates achieving a high enough score in Stage 2. At the selection centre, candidates are assessed in a variety of tasks, such as a patient simulation exercise, group exercise and written prioritisation exercise.

    Stages 1–3 of the assessment process are blue-printed against the national person specification[1] which is itself based on Good Medical Practice.[2]

- Stage 4 (allocation and offer) follows for successful candidates. The candidates who scored the highest in Stage 3 and the relevant parts of Stage 2 are most likely to be offered the programmes of their choice. If a deanery cannot offer a post to a suitable candidate, the candidate can be offered a post at another deanery via the national clearing process of the National Recruitment Office.

REFERENCES

1. http://www.gprecruitment.org.uk

2. General Medical Council. *Good Medical Practice (2006)*. Available at www.gmc-uk.org/guidance/good_medical_practice

Clinical Problem
Solving Questions

INTRODUCTION TO CLINICAL PROBLEM SOLVING QUESTIONS

The purpose of GP training is to provide the trainee with the necessary competences to practise independently as a general practitioner (http://www.rcgp-curriculum.org.uk), not to thrust knowledge into an individual. However, a candidate is expected, after 5–6 years as a medical student and 2 years as a foundation doctor, to have a reasonable level of knowledge and to be able to apply it to clinical situations. This is what the first part of Stage 2 assesses.

The assessment consists of a 75-minute question paper. The questions are in the form of clinical scenarios that require candidates to exercise judgement and problem solving skills to determine the appropriate diagnosis and management of patients. The level of difficulty of the questions will be such that a year 2 foundation programme doctor could reasonably be expected to answer. Thus, none of the questions requires specific knowledge about general practice.

The questions are evenly distributed across specific topic areas:

- Cardiovascular
- Dermatology/ENT/eye
- Endocrinology/metabolic
- Gastroenterology/nutrition
- Infectious disease/haematology/immunology/genetics
- Musculoskeletal
- Paediatrics
- Pharmacology/therapeutics
- Psychiatry/neurology
- Renal/urology
- Reproductive (male and female)
- Respiratory

Questions will relate to:

- Disease factors
- Making a diagnosis
- Investigations
- Management
- Prescribing
- Emergency care

The questions may appear in a variety of formats but two formats are commonly used, Extending Matching Questions and Single Best Answer Questions. In both formats, candidates have to choose the most likely of the given possible responses to a question, according to their clinical judgement. Unless otherwise stated, only one answer is required. It will often be an answer that could be found in a nationally approved guideline or the *British National Formulary*. Other answers may be plausible, but one will clearly be the most appropriate.

A sample Extending Matching Question and Single Best Answer Question are given overleaf.

EXTENDED MATCHING QUESTION

In Extending Matching Questions, a number of scenarios relating to a 'theme' are matched to the most appropriate choice from a list of options.

Example

THEME: FEBRILE CHILDREN

A Chickenpox

B Erythema infectiosum

C Hand, foot and mouth disease

D Herpangina

E Herpes simplex

F Rubella

G Scarlet fever

H Vincent angina

For each clinical scenario given below, select the single most likely diagnosis from the list above. Each option may be selected once, more than once or not at all.

☐ 1   A 4-year-old boy is pyrexial and has a sore throat and an erythematous rash that spares the area around the mouth. The tongue is red with prominent papillae.

☐ 2   A 5-year-old girl has been unwell for 2 days. She now has oedematous erythematous plaques on the cheeks.

☐ 3   A 3-year-old girl has a sore mouth with diffuse ulceration. She is dripping saliva and there are vesicles around her mouth.

☐ 4   A 2-year-old boy develops crops of vesicles on an erythematous base on the head, body and arms. The crops appear in different stages. There are ulcers in the mouth.

Answers

1   **G** Scarlet fever

2   **B** Erythema infectiosum

3   **E** Herpes simplex

4   **A** Chickenpox

SINGLE BEST ANSWER QUESTION

Single Best Answer Questions consist of a statement followed by a number of items, *one* of which is correct.

Example

1   **A 34-year-old woman returns 7 days after receiving chloramphenicol eye drops for apparent conjunctivitis. Her eyes feel gritty and water. There is diffuse infection of the sclera.**

         Select the single most likely diagnosis from the list below.

☐   **A**   Bacterial conjunctivitis

☐   **B**   Episcleritis

☐   **C**   Iritis

☐   **D**   Keratitis

☐   **E**   Viral conjunctivitis

Answer   E   Viral conjunctivitis

Occasionally, more than one answer may be required (Multiple Best Answer Question) so it is important to read each question carefully. Beside clinical scenarios, results of investigations may also be presented. Photographs or electrocardiograms may also be included.

Each correct answer is awarded one mark and the total score equals the number of correct answers. The score required to proceed to Stage 3 varies from year to year and depends on many factors, not least of which is how hard the paper is thought to be. This implies that a few hard questions can be expected. The purpose of the test is to distinguish between high and low achieving candidates and if all the questions are easy that task will be much more difficult. A few of the examples in this book are in the difficult category for the same reason.

There is no negative marking in this test (ie the loss of a mark when an incorrect answer is given). This removes the 'fear factor'. Candidates should pace themselves carefully and not run out of time. Where an answer is not known an intelligent guess should be made. No questions should be left unanswered as this may artificially lower the mark.

A lot of thought is given to the wording of the questions to try to make them as unambiguous as possible. However, it is important that candidates understand the meaning of certain conventional terms which frequently appear in the paper. These will be provided with the paper and can be found on the National Recruitment Office website. They are reproduced below and may appear in some of the questions in this book.

- *Pathognomonic, diagnostic, characteristic* and *in the vast majority* imply that a feature would occur in at least 90% of cases.

- *Typically, frequently, significantly, commonly* and *in a substantial majority* imply that a feature would occur in at least 60% of cases.

- *In the majority* implies that a feature occurs in greater than 50% of cases.

- *In the minority* implies that a feature occurs in less than 50% of cases.

- *Low chance* and *in a substantial minority* imply that a feature may occur in up to 30% of cases.

- *Has been shown, recognised* and *reported* all refer to evidence that can be found in authoritative medical texts. None of these terms make any implication about the frequency with which the feature occurs.

Candidates who do not already do so should start reading thoroughly. Review articles and editorials in major journals are useful. Weaknesses in the minor specialties can be covered by reading books such as the *ABC of Dermatology* and the *ABC of Eyes* (both published by BMJ Publishing Group). It is useful to be aware of the main conclusions presented in the different sections of *Clinical Evidence* (BMJ Publishing Group; www.clinicalevidence. com). A good working knowledge of the *British National Formulary* will be invaluable. Lastly, there is no substitute for seeing plenty of patients and reflecting on the diagnostic and management issues presented, and the effect of the illness on a patient's life.

Chapter 1
Cardiovascular

QUESTIONS

THEME: CHEST PAIN

Options

A Coronary artery spasm

B Dissection of thoracic aorta

C Gastro-oesophageal reflux disease

D Mesothelioma

E Metastatic lung deposits

F Oesophageal spasm

G Pericarditis

H Pneumonia

I Pneumothorax

J Pulmonary embolism

K Tietze disease

L Unstable angina

From each of the case scenarios given below, select the single most appropriate diagnosis from the above list of options. Each option may be used once, more than once or not at all.

☐ **1.1** A 25-year-old man has central chest pain, tachycardia and sweating. He has taken cocaine.

☐ **1.2** A 63-year-old male smoker has long-term hypertension. He has severe chest pain radiating to his back.

☐ **1.3** A 37-year-old woman has severe left-sided pain, which is worse on inspiration. She has antiphospholipid syndrome and a swollen left ankle.

☐ **1.4** A 42-year-old man has central chest pain. Movement exacerbates the pain and the anterior chest wall is tender.

☐ **1.5** A 67-year-old male industrial worker has left-sided chest pain and long-term pleural plaques.

☐ **1.6** An obese 42-year-old woman has central chest pain going through to her back, and this is worse in bed.

THEME: BASIC LIFE SUPPORT MANAGEMENT

Options

A   Check airway

B   Check pulse

C   Continue cardiopulmonary resuscitation (CPR) until exhausted

D   Give rescue breaths

E   Leave patient

F   No action

G   Place in recovery position

H   Start chest compressions

For each of the patients below, choose the single most appropriate treatment from the list of options above. Each option may be used once, more than once or not at all.

☐ **1.7**   A 6-year-old has stopped breathing in the supermarket. You have given mouth-to-mouth ventilation. What do you do next?

☐ **1.8**   A 73-year-old male visitor collapses in the hospital shop. You are the only other person in the shop. You open his airway and find he is not breathing.

☐ **1.9**   A 43-year-old man collapses in the street. After you open his airway he starts groaning.

☐ **1.10**   You rescue a 17-year-old boy from under the water in a canal. He is in cardiac arrest. You perform cardiopulmonary resuscitation alone for 1 minute and stop to assess your next action. The patient is unresponsive and cold.

☐ **1.11**   There has been a bomb blast at a London underground train station and the man in the seat next to you has stopped breathing. The train is full of black smoke and you can see a fire.

THEME: DRUGS USED IN CARDIOLOGY

Options

A	Amlodipine	G	Lisinopril
B	Atorvastatin	H	Losartan
C	Clopidogrel	I	Sotalol
D	Digoxin	J	Spironolactone
E	Dipyridamole	K	Warfarin
F	Furosemide		

For each patient described below, choose the single most appropriate treatment from the above list of options. Each option may be used once, more than once or not at all.

☐ **1.12** A 70-year-old man has stable angina and hypertension. His medication consists of aspirin, ramipril and simvastatin. He develops a weakness in his left arm and leg that resolves within 24 hours. His blood pressure is 135/85 and his pulse 78 and regular.

☐ **1.13** A 75-year-old woman has a troublesome cough six weeks after discharge from hospital where her heart failure was treated. Her medication includes bisoprolol, and ramipril.

☐ **1.14** The same woman's cough settles but she remains moderately dyspnoeic. There is no obvious evidence of fluid retention and her pulse is 88 and regular.

☐ **1.15** A 50-year-old woman has had two visits to the Emergency Department because she had atrial fibrillation. On both occasions she reverted to sinus rhythm.

☐ **1.16** An 80-year-old man has symptoms of angina on exertion but has declined invasive investigations. There has been some symptom improvement with oral and sub-lingual nitrates and atenolol but he still finds the angina troublesome.

THEME: PREVENTION OF CARDIOVASCULAR DISEASE

Options

A ACE inhibitor
B Aspirin
C β-blocker
D Calcium channel blocker
E Ezetimbe
F Fibrate
G Lifestyle advice only
H No treatment needed
I Statin

For each patient below, choose the single most suitable option from the above list for cardiovascular disease prevention. Each option may be used once, more than once or not at all.

☐ 1.17 A 48-year-old woman has recently been diagnosed with type 2 diabetes and is found to have a fasting total cholesterol level of 4.9mmol/l and triglyceride of 2.0mmol/l.

☐ 1.18 A 50-year-old man has an average blood pressure of 165/100 after serial measurements. His cholesterol is 4.0mmol/l and random blood sugar 5.0mmol/l. He is a non-smoker and has no family history of cardiovascular disease.

☐ 1.19 A 52-year-old man takes ramipril to control his blood pressure. The current measurement is 130/80.

☐ 1.20 A 70-year-old man has had an exercise ECG that is suggestive of coronary heart disease and is awaiting further investigations. His current medication includes aspirin, atenolol, bendroflumethiazide, and simvastatin. His last three blood pressure readings average is 150/95.

☐ 1.21 An otherwise healthy 40-year-old woman smokes 10 cigarettes per day. Her blood pressure is 120/80, total cholesterol 4.2mmol/l, LDL cholesterol 2.0mmol/l and random blood sugar 5.5mmol/l. Her cardiovascular disease risk is estimated at less than 10% over the next 10 years.

THEME: CLINICAL SIGNS OF STRUCTURAL HEART ABNORMALITIES

Options

A	Atrial septal defect	**H**	Mitral stenosis
B	Aortic incompetence	**I**	Mitral valve prolapse
C	Aortic sclerosis	**J**	Patent ductus arteriosus
D	Aortic stenosis	**K**	Pulmonary stenosis
E	Hypertrophic cardiomyopathy	**L**	Tricuspid regurgitation
F	Left ventricular aneurysm	**M**	Tricuspid stenosis
G	Mitral incompetence	**N**	Ventricular septal defect (VSD)

For each description of clinical signs below, choose the single most likely diagnosis from the list of options above. Each option may be used once, more than once or not at all.

☐ **1.22** There is a harsh pan-systolic murmur, loudest at the lower left sternal edge and inaudible at the apex. The apex is not displaced.

☐ **1.23** There is a soft late systolic murmur at the apex, radiating to the axilla.

☐ **1.24** The pulse is slow rising and the apex, which is not displaced, is heaving in character. There is an ejection systolic murmur heard best at the right second interspace that does not radiate.

☐ **1.25** The pulse is regular and jerky in character. The cardiac impulse is hyperdynamic and not displaced. There is a mid-systolic murmur, with no ejection click, loudest at the left sternal edge.

☐ **1.26** There is a constant 'machinery-like' murmur throughout systole and diastole.

THEME: CARDIOLOGY IN CHILDREN

Options

A Admit immediately to a paediatric unit
B Chest X-ray
C Electrocardiogram
D Follow-up appointment
E Ignore the findings
F Routine outpatient appointment

For each of the patients below, choose the single most appropriate management option from the list of options above. Each option may be used once, more than once or not at all.

☐ **1.27** A 6-year-old visits her GP with fever and earache. On examination she looks well but is febrile and has otitis media. It is also noted that there is a quiet systolic murmur localised to the left sternal edge. Otherwise cardiac examination is normal.

☐ **1.28** A 6-week-old baby presents with difficulty feeding and poor weight gain. On examination the baby is tachypnoeic and tachycardic. There is a loud systolic murmur, intercostal recession and hepatomegaly.

☐ **1.29** A 3-day-old baby presents to the Emergency Department with central cyanosis. There is a systolic murmur but otherwise the cardiovascular examination is normal.

☐ **1.30** During a routine 8-week baby check, the GP hears a loud pansystolic murmur at the left sternal edge. Otherwise the examination is normal and the baby is asymptomatic and thriving.

1.31   A 60-year-old man has crushing central chest pain of one hour duration.

Select from the list below the single measure that would not be appropriate prior to recording an ECG.

- [ ] **A**   Aspirin 300mg chewed
- [ ] **B**   Cyclizine intra venous 50mg
- [ ] **C**   Glyceryl trinitrate sublingually
- [ ] **D**   Diamorphine intravenous 5mg
- [ ] **E**   Tenecteplase intravenous 50mg

1.32   A 72-year-old man has heart failure and chronic obstructive pulmonary disease (COPD). He has come for his medication to be reviewed. His current medications are aspirin, lisinopril, simvastatin and inhalers for his COPD.

Which one other medication would he most benefit from?

- [ ] **A**   Amlodipine
- [ ] **B**   Bisoprolol
- [ ] **C**   Digoxin
- [ ] **D**   Losartan
- [ ] **E**   Ramipril

1.33 A 63-year-old woman with hypertension and recently diagnosed thyrotoxicosis complains of recent-onset palpitations. She is worried that the new medication she is taking for her thyrotoxicosis is causing these symptoms.

Which one of the following is the single most likely diagnosis in this patient?

- ☐ **A** Atrial fibrillation
- ☐ **B** Heart block
- ☐ **C** Heart failure
- ☐ **D** Side-effect of carbimazole
- ☐ **E** Ventricular ectopics

1.34 A patient is newly diagnosed with atrial fibrillation.

Select the single feature from the list below that would make the decision to prescribe aspirin rather than warfarin more appropriate.

- ☐ **A** Age > 75 years
- ☐ **B** Age < 65 years
- ☐ **C** Aortic stenosis
- ☐ **D** Heart failure
- ☐ **E** Previous transient ischaemic attack

1.35   A 78-year-old woman presents with dyspnoea. Her pulse is regular but there are alternating weak and strong beats.

Select from the list below the single condition that this type of pulse is characteristic of.

☐ **A**   Aortic regurgitation
☐ **B**   Aortic stenosis
☐ **C**   Cardiac tamponade
☐ **D**   Severe left ventricular failure
☐ **E**   Takayasu's arteritis

ANSWERS

THEME: CHEST PAIN

1.1   A   Coronary artery spasm

Cocaine causes agitation, tachycardia, hypertension, arrhythmias and coronary artery spasm. Coronary artery spasm may lead to angina-type chest pain and even myocardial infarction.

1.2   B   Dissection of thoracic aorta

Dissection of the aorta within the chest causes severe central pain, that usually radiates to the back between the scapulae. Dissection of the aorta is associated with hypertension and collagen disorders (Marfan syndrome, pseudoxanthoma elasticum). Late-stage syphilis is also associated with dissection.

1.3   J   Pulmonary embolism

A clot has embolised from this lady's leg and her lung is infarcted. Antiphospholipid antibody syndrome is an autoimmune disorder that predisposes to recurrent thromboses. The clinical presentation of pulmonary embolism ranges from mild pleuritic chest pain to cardiac arrest. Patients are often mildly short of breath and hypoxic on arterial blood gas testing and D-dimer testing will be positive. Chest X-rays are often normal. Diagnosis is by ventilation/perfusion scanning or spiral computed tomography.

1.4   K   Tietze disease

This disorder is caused by inflammation around the costosternal junctions. It may be bilateral or unilateral and the chest wall is very tender over the affected area. Reassurance and non-steroidal anti-inflammatory drugs (NSAIDs) are the mainstays of treatment.

1.5   D   Mesothelioma

This patient has long-standing pleural plaques, a sign of major previous asbestos exposure. Asbestos has many adverse effects on the lung, including pleural thickening (plaques), pleural effusions, fibrosis and mesothelioma. It is also associated with carcinoma of the bronchus. No medical treatment is known to alter the progress of asbestos-related disease.

1.6   C   Gastro-oesophageal reflux disease

This woman has reflux of gastric contents into the oesophagus, the acid nature of which is irritating the oesophageal mucosa and causing pain. This is often an indigestion-type pain, which may be relieved by antacids or proton pump inhibitors. Obesity, fatty foods, alcohol, cigarette smoking and large meals are associated with symptomatic disease. Complications include oesophageal stricture and Barrett oesophagus.

THEME: BASIC LIFE SUPPORT MANAGEMENT

1.7   B   Check pulse

In a cardiac arrest in a child, the recommendation is first to open the airway, then to check breathing. If the child is not breathing, five effective rescue breaths are given. After this, a central pulse should be checked. If this is absent then external cardiac massage is started. Alternate between cardiac massage and breaths at a ratio of 15:2 for two trained personnel, or 30:2 for lone rescuer. Continue for 1 minute. After this obtain access to advanced life support. You may be able to carry the child to a telephone if no one else has summoned help. In reality, in a supermarket help will be on its way. In this case you continue CPR until help arrives or you become exhausted.[1]

1.8   E   Leave patient

The most likely cause of a respiratory arrest in this adult patient is a cardiac arrest. The best chance of a successful outcome is if the patient is in ventricular fibrillation and is electrically defibrillated. In this situation you should leave the patient to summon help before starting basic life support.[1]

1.9   G   Place in recovery position

Groaning implies return of spontaneous breathing, and also adequate circulation. However, the man has a reduced level of consciousness. If he is lying on his back there is a danger of the tongue blocking the airway so he should be placed in the recovery position.

1.10   E   Leave patient

Rescue from drowning is an indication to start CPR rather than leaving the patient to summon help and a defibrillator. If there has been no response to initial CPR, leave the patient to get help. In an adult who may have sustained trauma or whose condition indicates drowning as the cause of cardiac arrest, the first action is also to give 1 minute of CPR prior to leaving to summon help.[1]

1.11   E   Leave patient

Your own safety is at risk. There is no merit in becoming another victim.

THEME: DRUGS USED IN CARDIOLOGY

1.12   E   Dipyridamole

NICE recommends[2] that a combination of modified-release dipyridamole and aspirin be used to prevent occlusive vascular events in those who have had a transient ischaemic attack (as with this patient) or an ischaemic stroke. The combination should be used for 2 years after the last event and the low dose aspirin continued thereafter. Warfarin is likely to be used instead if this patient had atrial fibrillation.

1.13   H   Losartan

Losartan (an angiotensin II receptor antagonist) should be substituted for the ACE inhibitor ramipril. Troublesome dry cough is a common side effect with ACE inhibitors. Unfortunately losartan can also produce cough. β-blockers can cause wheezing and that can make patients cough.

1.14   J   Spironolactone

Current guidelines[3] recommend that patients already on optimal doses of a β-blocker and ACE inhibitor should have an aldosterone antagonist, spironolactone added to their therapy. Furosemide is used to control congestive symptoms and fluid retention. Digoxin can be used if she remains symptomatic in spite of the above therapy or if she has atrial fibrillation.

1.15   I   Sotalol

There is a wide choice of antiarrhythmic agents to prevent the recurrence of atrial fibrillation. The β-blocker sotalol is commonly used. In fact its licence is limited to the management of ventricular arrhythmias and the prophylaxis of supraventricular arrhythmias. β-blockers are also used to control heart rate in patients with persistent atrial fibrillation. Digoxin is an alternative rate control drug for such patients.

1.16   A   Amlodipine

For symptom control in angina the addition of a calcium channel blocker is the next step. Nicorandil, a potassium channel activator might also help. He should take aspirin if tolerated and any risk factors should be managed appropriately. He should have as full a clinical assessment as he will permit and exacerbating factors such as anaemia should be excluded.

THEME: PREVENTION OF CARDIOVASCULAR DISEASE

These questions and answers are based on the Joint British Societies' guidelines on the prevention of cardiovascular disease in clinical practice.[4]

1.17   I   Statin

Cholesterol lowering therapy (statins) should be prescribed for all people with type 1 or 2 diabetes who are over the age of 40 years. Younger patients with other risk factors, poor diabetic control, complications or a cholesterol level > 6.0mmol/l should also be given a statin.

1.18   A   ACE inhibitor

Healthy people should receive lifestyle advice and drug therapy if the blood pressure is sustained at levels of 160/100 or greater regardless of the absolute level of cardiovascular risk. Treatment targets are to produce levels of 140/85 or less. An ACE inhibitor is the recommended treatment for a patient under the age of 55 years.[5]

1.19   B   Aspirin

Aspirin 75mg daily should be prescribed for hypertensive patients over the age of 50 years whose blood pressure is controlled to a level of 150/90 or less.

1.20   A   ACE inhibitor

ACE inhibitors are recommended for patients with ischaemic heart disease particularly if there is reduced left ventricular function. They should also be considered for patients with normal left ventricular function if the blood pressure targets have not been achieved (< 130/80 in patients with ischaemic heart disease). Other risk factors need attention and the statin dose may need adjustment. Aspirin and a β-blocker, both beneficial, are already being taken.

1.21   G   Lifestyle advice only

Cardiovascular risk estimation charts use the risk factors: gender, cholesterol:HDL cholesterol ratio, diabetes, smoking and systolic blood pressure. Healthy individuals with a cardiovascular disease risk of < 20% over 10 years and no cardiovascular complications or diabetes should receive lifestyle advice and be reassessed in 5 years.

THEME: CLINICAL SIGNS OF STRUCTURAL HEART ABNORMALITIES

1.22   N   Ventricular septal defect

The amplitude of a murmur depends on the amount of turbulence or flow. A small VSD (maladie de Roger) is louder than a large one. With a small VSD the pressure in the left ventricle is higher than the right so there is high flow per cross-sectional area of the defect. In a large VSD, ventricular pressures may equalise and there will be no flow across the defect. Reversal of the direction of flow (ie a right-to-left shunt) may occur, precipitating cyanosis and breathlessness. This is Eisenmenger syndrome and may occur acutely or chronically.

1.23   I   Mitral valve prolapse

Late systolic murmurs that otherwise resemble mitral incompetence are usually due to mitral valve prolapse but may also be due to mild mitral incompetence (usually secondary to prolapse in such cases). There may also (or only) be a mid-systolic click. Clinical identification is important, as most cardiologists advise endocarditis prophylaxis for patients with mitral valve prolapse if it is clinically apparent, but not if it is an echo-only diagnosis.

1.24   D   Aortic stenosis

This is the classic description of aortic stenosis. As the gradient increases the murmur gets louder and the pulse pressure becomes lower. There may also be postural hypotension. As the left ventricle fails, however, the murmur becomes softer as the flow through the valve is reduced.

1.25   E   Hypertrophic cardiomyopathy

This is a classic description of hypertrophic cardiomyopathy. The hypertrophic septum causes functional obstruction of the left ventricular outflow tract (subaortic stenosis) and produces a murmur similar to aortic stenosis except that the second heart sound is normal.

1.26   J   Patent ductus arteriosus

Patent ductus arteriosus is now almost always identified and treated in the neonatal period. The murmur, when heard, is usually characteristic.

THEME: CARDIOLOGY IN CHILDREN

1.27   D   Follow-up appointment

This is likely to be an innocent murmur, which up to a third of children have at some point. They are not associated with any structural abnormality. The features of an innocent murmur are a quiet systolic murmur at the left sternal edge with no radiation. There is no diastolic component and no thrill. The child is otherwise asymptomatic and thriving. These murmurs are common during a febrile illness, due to the increased cardiac output.

1.28   A   Admit immediately to a paediatric unit

This baby has signs and symptoms suggestive of heart failure. The other common symptoms are sweating and recurrent chest infections. This baby needs an urgent assessment by a paediatrician. An electrocardiogram (ECG) and chest X-ray may help with diagnosing the underlying cause.

1.29   A   Admit immediately to a paediatric unit

This baby may have a duct-dependent cardiac defect. When the ductus arteriosus closes in the first few days of life the baby will become symptomatic, and survival will then balance on maintaining the patency of the duct with prostaglandin. This is a paediatric emergency and the baby needs to be assessed urgently by a paediatrician.

1.30   F   Routine outpatient appointment

This baby may have a ventricular septal defect. This is the commonest congenital heart defect. It is often picked up incidentally at a routine examination. The defect often closes spontaneously in the first week of life. As the baby is well they can be seen in an outpatient clinic. For the meantime, you should tell the parents about the signs of heart failure and to seek help if they occur.

1.31   E   Tenecteplase intravenous 50mg

Thrombolytic therapy is the accepted treatment for acute ST elevation myocardial infarction and should be given at the earliest opportunity. It is indicated if there is a strong clinical suspicion of myocardial infarction and the pain is unrelieved by nitrate and there is an unequivocally abnormal ECG (normally at least 1mm ST elevation in two limb leads or at least 2mm in any two adjacent chest leads or new onset left bundle branch block).[6] Whether treatment is started in hospital or in the community will depend on geographical location and local guidelines. Aspirin and nitrate should be given unless contraindicated. Analgesia and an anti-emetic may be needed to help stabilise the patient.

1.32   B   Bisoprolol

COPD is not an absolute contraindication to β-blocker treatment. In cases where up-titration is difficult, results from studies indicated that in terms of mortality and symptoms, some β-blocker is better than no β-blocker. Sometimes initiation of β-blockers is done in secondary care so the patient may need to be referred back to the hospital for this. Temporary exacerbation of symptoms may occur in 20–30% of patients when treatment with β-blockers is started, which may require increasing the dose of diuretic treatment.

1.33   A   Atrial fibrillation

Atrial fibrillation is the most likely cause of this patient's palpitations. Thyrotoxicosis can precipitate atrial fibrillation. It is important that she is given medication to control the heart rate, and anticoagulation should be considered. As the thyrotoxicosis improves, the atrial fibrillation may well improve or the patient may even revert back to sinus rhythm.

1.34   B   Age < 65 years

NICE clinical guidelines[7] include a stroke risk stratification algorithm. All the options except that of age less than 65 years predict a high risk of stroke. Warfarin is more beneficial in stroke prevention but its use involves regular monitoring of INR levels making it more time consuming for patients. Patients less than 65 years without other risk factors are in a low risk group and NICE suggests that aspirin is a reasonable option. The difficult group is between the ages of 65 years and 75 years, particularly if moderate risk factors such as diabetes, hypertension and vascular disease are present. Here the physician must balance the risk benefits of the two drugs. As stroke risk factors are cumulative, the presence of two might sway the physician in favour of warfarin. Informed consent on the part of the patient is particularly relevant here.

1.35   D   Severe left ventricular failure

This is pulsus alternans and describes a pulse with a regular rhythm but with alternating weak and strong beats. It is found in patients with severe heart failure and suggests a poor prognosis, ie prolonged recovery of the failing heart muscles.

REFERENCES

1. Resuscitation Council (UK). *The Resuscitation Guidelines* (homepage on the Internet), 2005 (updated 2007 August; cited 2008 April 23). Available from http://www.resus.org.uk/pages/guide.htm

2. National Institute for Health and Clinical Excellence. *Clopidogrel and modified-release dipyridamole in the prevention of occlusive vascular events.* (homepage on the Internet), May 2005 (cited 2008 April 23). Available from http://www.nice.org.uk/nicemedia/pdf/ TA090guidance.pdf

3. National Institute for Health and Clinical Excellence, Clinical Guidelines 5. *Management of chronic heart failure in adults in primary and secondary care events.* (homepage on the Internet), July 2003 (cited 2008 April 23). Available from http://www.nice.org.uk/nicemedia/pdf/ CG5NICEguideline.pdf

4. Wood D, Wray R, Poulter N et al. *Joint British Societies guidelines on prevention of cardiovascular disease in clinical practice.* Heart 2005: 91 (supplement 5): v1–v52

5. National Institute for Health and Clinical Excellence. *Hypertension: management of hypertension of adults in primary care.* (homepage on the Internet), June 2006 (cited 2008 April 23). Available from http:// www.nice.org.uk/CG034

6. Scottish Heart and Arterial Disease Risk Prevention. *Brief guidelines for general practitioners giving thrombolytic therapy.* 2001.

7. National Institute for Health and Clinical Excellence. *Atrial fibrillation: the management of atrial fibrillation.* Quick reference guide (homepage on the Internet), June 2006 (cited 2008 April 23). Available from http:// www.nice.org.uk/nicemedia/pdf/CG036quickrefguide.pdf

Chapter 2
Dermatology, ENT and Eye

QUESTIONS

THEME: ACUTE RED EYE

Options

A Acute glaucoma
B Central retinal vein occlusion
C Conjunctivitis
D Dacryocystitis
E Episcleritis

F Iritis
G Keratitis
H Scleritis
I Subconjunctival haemorrhage

For each of the clinical scenarios below, choose the single most likely diagnosis from the list of options above. Each option may be used once, more than once or not at all.

☐ **2.1** A 20-year-old man has bilateral itchy red eyes with profuse watery discharge but with normal visual acuity. The tarsal conjunctiva reveals a follicular appearance.

☐ **2.2** A 30-year-old woman has a painful red eye with a mucopurulent discharge. There is circumcorneal redness, with a hypopyon and opacity of the cornea.

☐ **2.3** A 40-year-old man has a red left eye with pain, photophobia and mild reduction in visual acuity, and a small pupil.

☐ **2.4** A 75-year-old man has a severely painful red eye with reduced visual acuity, nausea and vomiting. The pupil is fixed and semi-dilated. There is intense engorgement of the corneal and episcleral vessels with corneal oedema.

☐ **2.5** A 35-year-old woman has acute painful erythema limited to the inferolateral quadrant of the right eye.

THEME: RETINAL EXAMINATION

Options

A   Age-related macular degeneration

B   Benign intracranial hypertension

C   Central retinal vein occlusion

D   Cytomegalovirus retinitis

E   Hypertensive retinopathy

F   Non-proliferative diabetic retinopathy

G   Proliferative diabetic retinopathy

H   Retinal artery occlusion

For each of the patients below study the retinal image and choose the single most likely diagnosis from the list of options above. Each option may be used once, more than once or not at all.

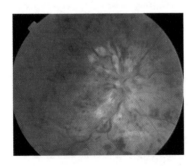

☐ **2.6**   This 71-year-old man reports sudden deterioration of vision in the right eye. His blood pressure is 180/100.

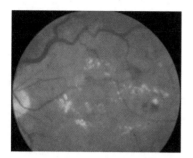

☐ **2.7** This 58-year-old woman has a blood pressure of 160/100 and a body mass index of 31.

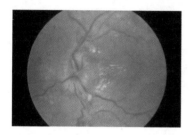

☐ **2.8** This 62-year-old woman reports sudden deterioration in vision in the left eye. Her blood pressure is 165/110 and her pulse is 100 and irregular.

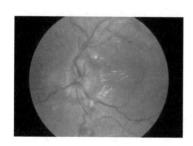

☐ **2.9** This 32-year-old man complains of intermittent headaches over the past three months. His blood pressure is 240/125.

THEME: DIAGNOSIS OF RASHES

Options

A	Bullous pemphigoid	G	Necrobiosis lipoidica
B	Dermatitis herpetiformis	H	Pemphigus vulgaris
C	Erythema nodosum	I	Psoriasis
D	Herpes simplex	J	Vasculitis
E	Herpes zoster	K	Vitiligo
F	Lichen planus	L	Warts

For each of the patients below study the photograph and choose the single most likely diagnosis from the list of options above. Each option may be used once, more than once or not at all.

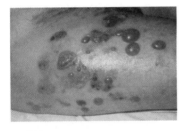

☐ **2.10** This 56-year-old woman has painless blisters, mainly on the lower limbs but also some on the trunk.

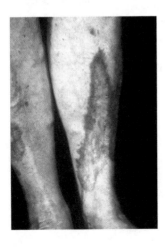

☐ **2.11** This 42-year-old woman has noticed a rash on both lower limbs, which has slowly extended.

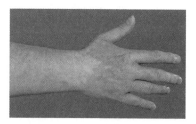

☐ **2.12** This 55-year-old woman is undergoing investigation for anaemia. Her haemoglobin is 9.8g/dl and mean cell volume 118fl. She shows you her hands but has similar lesions elsewhere.

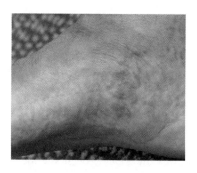

☐ **2.13** This 50-year-old man has slightly itchy papules on the medial aspect of both feet. There are a few lesions at the wrists and ankles.

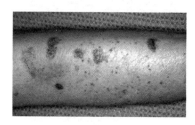

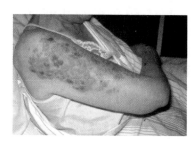

☐ **2.14** This 56-year-old man shows you these lesions that are mainly on his lower legs and are just palpable when you run your finger along them.

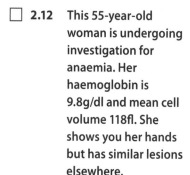

☐ **2.15** This 58-year-old woman developed this painful rash on her right arm four days ago.

THEME: TOPICAL THERAPY IN DERMATOLOGY

Options

A Acne vulgaris

B Atopic eczema

C Herpes zoster

D Hyperhidrosis

E Molluscum contagiosum

F Pityriasis versicolor

G Plantar wart

H Psoriasis

I Rosacea

J Scabies

For each of the topical treatments listed below choose the single most appropriate indication from the list of options above. Each option may be used once, more than once or not at all.

☐ **2.16** Benzoyl peroxide 5% in aqueous gel

☐ **2.17** Calcipotriol cream

☐ **2.18** Clobetasone butyrate 1% ointment

☐ **2.19** Clotrimazole 1% cream

☐ **2.20** Permethrin 1% cream

☐ **2.21** Salicylic acid 16.7%, lactic acid 16.7% in flexible colloidon

THEME: DEAFNESS

Options

A	Acoustic neuroma	**F**	Noise induced deafness
B	Acute otitis externa	**G**	Otitis media with effusion
C	Acute otitis media	**H**	Otosclerosis
D	Chronic suppurative otitis media	**I**	Presbyacusis
		J	Stroke
E	Ménière's disease	**K**	Wax

For each patient below, choose the single most likely diagnosis from the list of options above. Each option may be used once, more than once or not at all.

☐ **2.22** A 65-year-old man's hearing has gradually deteriorated. It is worse in a noisy environment. Both ears are involved and Rinne's test is positive. The ear drums look normal.

☐ **2.23** A 55-year-old man has a gradual onset of deafness and tinnitus in the left ear. The ear drum looks normal and Rinne's test is positive.

☐ **2.24** Following a visit to a swimming pool a 38-year-old man has mild discomfort and deafness in his left ear. A solid plug of material prevents visualisation of the ear drum.

☐ **2.25** A 32-year-old woman's hearing loss that has worsened during her recent pregnancy. Both ears are involved and Rinne's test is negative. The ear drums look normal.

☐ **2.26** A 49-year-old woman has longstanding hearing loss in the right ear. She has had ear discharge in the past and once again it is offensive. There is a central perforation of the eardrum.

THEME: INVESTIGATION OF LUMPS IN THE NECK

Options

A Doppler ultrasound

B Digital subtraction angiography

C Excision biopsy

D Fine needle aspiration

E Iodine uptake scan

F Nasopharyngoscopy

G Paul Bunnell test

H Sialogram

I Technetium scan

J Thyroid function tests

K Ultrasound

For each of the patients below, choose the most discriminatory investigation from the list of options above. Each option may be used once, more than once or not at all.

☐ **2.27** A 53-year-old woman presents with a 6-month history of a mass below the angle of the jaw on the right. It is gradually increasing in size and is mobile and firm to the touch. There is no associated pain or facial weakness.

☐ **2.28** A 68-year-old man presents with a mass in the anterior triangle of the neck. It has increased in size over the past 2 months. It is soft, pulsatile and there is an associated bruit.

☐ **2.29** A 38-year-old woman presents with a 2-month history of a swelling in the anterior part of the neck, towards the left of the midline. The swelling is not painful and she feels otherwise well. On examination, she has a solitary thyroid nodule in the left lobe of the thyroid. She is clinically euthyroid.

CHAPTER 2 QUESTIONS

☐ **2.30** A 46-year-old woman presents with a diffuse swelling in the anterior part of the neck. She also complains of a hoarse voice. On examination, she has a diffuse multinodular goitre, bradycardia and slow-relaxing reflexes.

☐ **2.31** A 27-year-old man complains of an intermittent painful swelling below his jaw. The pain and swelling is worse on eating. He is otherwise well. On examination, there is a small, tender swelling in the left submandibular region.

☐ **2.32** A 72-year-old man presents with a hard, painless swelling in the anterior triangle of the neck. He has had a hoarse voice for 2 months. He is a lifelong smoker and drinks heavily.

CHAPTER 2 QUESTIONS

2.33 A 75-year-old woman has deteriorating vision. She also notices that when she looks at a straight line it appears wavy and part of the line is missing.

From the options below select the single most likely diagnosis.

- [ ] **A** Age-related macular degeneration
- [ ] **B** Cataract
- [ ] **C** Chronic glaucoma
- [ ] **D** Migraine
- [ ] **E** Temporal arteritis

2.34 A 70-year-old woman complains of a dark moving object in her right field of vision but no actual visual loss.

From the options below select the single most likely diagnosis.

- [ ] **A** Iritis
- [ ] **B** Migraine
- [ ] **C** Posterior vitreous detachment
- [ ] **D** Retinal detachment
- [ ] **E** Vitreous haemorrhage

2.35   This 65-year-old man presents with an itchy
erythematous rash involving both groins.

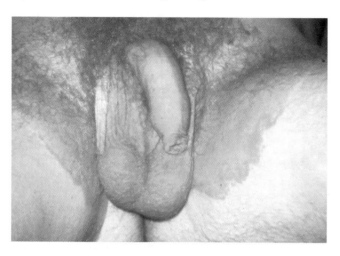

Which of the following is likely to be an effective treatment?

- **A**   Amoxycillin
- **B**   Chlorpheniramine
- **C**   Co-amoxiclav
- **D**   Hydrocortisone
- **E**   Miconazole

2.36 This 57-year-old woman is concerned about the appearance of her thumb.

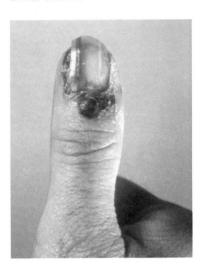

From the options below select the single most likely diagnosis.

- [ ] **A** Digital embolism
- [ ] **B** Malignant melanoma
- [ ] **C** Pyogenic granuloma
- [ ] **D** Subungual haematoma
- [ ] **E** Trauma

2.37 A 36-year-old man has had left sided facial pain with purulent nasal discharge for 10 days.

From the list below select the single treatment of choice.

- [ ] **A** Amoxycillin
- [ ] **B** Chlorpheniramine
- [ ] **C** Ephedrine
- [ ] **D** Flucloxacillin
- [ ] **E** Metronidazole

ANSWERS

THEME: ACUTE RED EYE

2.1   C   Conjunctivitis

In viral conjunctivitis there is a watery discharge with tarsal follicles.

2.2   G   Keratitis

The cornea is an avascular, transparent structure. A breach in the corneal epithelium is necessary for infection to become established. Bacterial infection is associated with a mucopurulent discharge. A hypopyon is seen when pus cells accumulate in the anterior chamber of the eye. The corneal opacity is the corneal ulcer. The most important viral keratitis is herpetic, with the formation of a dendritic ulcer, which can usually only be seen after fluorescein staining.

2.3   F   Iritis

This is acute iritis. The inflammation predominantly involves the iris and ciliary body. The pupil is smaller than the unaffected side. A hypopyon may be seen in severe cases in which keratic precipitates (aggregates of cells on the posterior surface of the cornea) will be visible on slit lamp examination.

2.4   A   Acute glaucoma

The main features of acute glaucoma are decreased vision associated with severe pain and constitutional upset. This condition is most commonly seen in older patients with long-sightedness. It is important to measure intraocular pressures and administer pupil-constricting eye drops, eg pilocarpine to open up the angle, as well as drugs such as acetazolamide to reduce the production of aqueous humour.

2.5   E   Episcleritis

Episcleritis is unilateral and frequently recurrent. It is more common in women aged 30–40 years. The redness is confined to one quadrant of the eye. A tender nodule may be present at the centre of the inflamed area. It may be associated with connective tissue disorders.

THEME: RETINAL EXAMINATION

2.6   C   Central retinal vein occlusion

There are extensive retinal haemorrhages and exudates involving all sectors of the retina. Central retinal vein occlusion is a thrombotic disorder (in contrast to central artery occlusion, which is usually embolic). Glaucoma is a risk factor. Branch retinal vein occlusion shows less retinal involvement.

2.7   F   Non-proliferative diabetic retinopathy

The obesity is a clue that this patient might be diabetic. The longer a patient has diabetes the greater the risk of retinopathy. The characteristic appearance includes microaneurysms (difficult to distinguish from dot haemorrhages), retinal haemorrhages and hard exudates that arise from increased capillary permeability and leakage of serum lipids and proteins. Co-existent hypertension makes progression to proliferative retinopathy and macular oedema more likely.

2.8   H   Retinal artery occlusion

The appearances indicate branch retinal artery occlusion (pallor and oedema). This presents with painless sudden onset unilateral visual field loss. The mechanism is usually embolic (eg carotid arteriosclerosis, atrial fibrillation), but may also be caused by temporal arteritis or suddenly increased intraocular pressure.

2.9   E   Hypertensive retinopathy

The appearances are typical of grade IV hypertensive retinopathy with exudates, haemorrhages and papilloedema. This indicates accelerated hypertension associated with severe end-organ damage and necessitates prompt treatment.

THEME: DIAGNOSIS OF RASHES

2.10   A   Bullous pemphigoid

Tense bullae are characteristic of pemphigoid. They rupture to leave erosions and crusts due to dried exudate. In bullous pemphigoid the split in the epidermis is at the level of the basement membrane and the blisters remain for a while before rupturing. This is in contrast to pemphigus where the intradermal split is higher in the epidermis so the bullae tend to rupture more easily. Involvement of mucous membranes is more common in pemphigus. Both are autoimmune conditions. In dermatitis herpetiformis there are papules, vesicles, small bullae, crusts and erosions grouped on an erythematous base. Most heavily involved are the elbows, the scapular, sacral and gluteal regions, and the knees. This condition is associated with gluten enteropathy and responds to a gluten-free diet. All these conditions are uncommon and bullae due to scalds, impetigo or insect bites are more frequently seen.

2.11   G   Necrobiosis lipoidica

Necrobiosis lipoidica (diabeticorum) is an idiopathic granulomatous disorder that typically occurs overlying the shins. Characteristic appearance is an erythematous patch with a yellowish hue that becomes progressively atrophic. Most patients with necrobiosis will have diabetes. Some of those who are not diabetic may get diabetes later. The association is with both the insulin-dependent and non-insulin-dependent types of diabetes. Only rarely does necrobiosis lipoidica clear up and this is not always the result of treatment (eg topical corticosteroids, psoralens and ultraviolet light), which is usually unsatisfactory.

2.12   K   Vitiligo

Vitiligo is an autoimmune disorder mediated by autoantibodies that target melanocytes resulting in patches of hypopigmentation. Patients are at risk of sunburn and skin cancer in affected sites in sun-exposed areas. It is associated with other autoimmune disorders including Graves' disease, hypoparathyroidism, insulin-dependent diabetes mellitus, Addison's disease, primary ovarian failures and, in this situation, pernicious anaemia. Treatment is unsatisfactory but, where it is disfiguring, cosmetic camouflage may give satisfactory results.

2.13   F   Lichen planus

Lichen planus is a papular disorder involving mainly skin and mucosa. Hair and nails may also be involved. The cause is not known. The papules are flat-topped and violaceous with white markings in a reticulate pattern (Wickham's striae). It is typically found on the flexor surfaces of the arms, the legs, genitalia, and sacrum. Papules commonly coalesce to form larger lesions. Scarring alopecia and nail fold destruction are recognised adverse effects. Topical corticosteroids will modify the inflammation. Resolving lesions are replaced by post-inflammatory hyperpigmentation.

2.14   J   Vasculitis

This man has palpable purpura, which is a sign of cutaneous vasculitis. Cutaneous vasculitis is a term for inflammation of the blood vessels in the skin. The inflammation can affect any of the vessels in the skin including capillaries, venules, arterioles and lymphatics. Cutaneous vasculitis can be due to any of several different causes including drugs, infections and autoimmune diseases, and can have a wide variety of clinical presentations. Larger areas of subcutaneous bleeding may be present or areas of skin may be necrotic. In more severe cases there may be systemic symptoms such as fever or joint pains. In most cases an underlying cause is not found and the disease is self-limiting. In a minority of patients, cutaneous vasculitis can be part of a more severe vasculitis affecting other organs.

2.15   E   Herpes zoster

Herpes zoster is often preceded by pain in the area to be affected. Then a rash of vesicles on a red background appears within a single dermatome. The lesions then crust. The site of the rash suggests C7 dermatome involvement. The chicken pox (varicella) virus is the causative organism. Lesions resolve in about 2 weeks. Pain may persist long after the lesions have resolved (post-herpetic neuralgia). Aciclovir can reduce the severity and duration of herpes zoster if a course is started within 72 hours of the appearance of the characteristic rash.

THEME: TOPICAL THERAPY IN DERMATOLOGY

2.16   A   Acne vulgaris

Benzoyl peroxide is useful in mild to moderate acne. Both comedones and inflamed lesions respond. It is applied once or twice a day. It may cause some erythema and peeling particularly at the start of treatment but this often settles. For this reason it is usual to start with a lower strength preparation before increasing frequency of application and strength gradually. Treatment is usually necessary for several months. It is often used in combination with topical retinoids and oral antibiotics in more severe acne.[1]

2.17   H   Psoriasis

Calcipotriol is a vitamin D analogue that affects cell division but has little effect on calcium metabolism. Because it does not smell or stain it is more acceptable than tar or dithranol and is now the first line treatment for chronic plaque psoriasis. Erythema, burning and itching are common side effects.[2]

2.18   B   Atopic eczema

Clobetasone butyrate is a topical corticosteroid, which along with emollients are the main preparations used to treat eczema. Topical corticosteroids are classified according to potency as mild, moderate, potent and very potent.[3] In general the mildest effective preparation for the condition should be used. For an infant with atopic eczema that would normally mean hydrocortisone 1%. Some types of eczema will require more potent corticosteroids. Clobetasone butyrate is classified as moderate in the potency table. It would be used where hydrocortisone is not effective or only slowly effective. A stepwise approach to treatment should be the rule so equally clobetasone butyrate could be used when stepping down from using the potent betametasone valerate 0.1%, for instance in the management of hand eczema or nummular eczema.

2.19   F   Pityriasis versicolor

This is a common skin disease caused by an overgrowth of the yeast fungus called *Malassezia furfur*. Sharply marginated oval macules of variable size occur most commonly on the upper back or chest. On un-tanned skin legions are light brown and on tanned skin white. There is fine scaling. A variety of agents are effective including azole creams and topical selenium sulphide.

2.20   J   Scabies

Treatment should be applied to the whole body including the scalp, neck, face and ears and left on overnight. All members of an affected household should be treated simultaneously. Two treatments should be applied a week apart. Itching may persist for several weeks after the infestation has been eliminated.

2.21   G   Plantar wart

Various salicylic acid preparations are available for the treatment of warts. Normally a daily application is made with measures to protect surrounding normal skin. The surface of the wart will need gentle filing with a pumice stone every few days. Treatment will need to be carried out for several weeks. Good research into the treatment of warts is scanty but a systematic review[4] showed cryotherapy not to be any more effective than salicylic acid. Cryotherapy has greater morbidity and is unacceptable to children.

THEME: DEAFNESS

2.22   I   Presbyacusis

This is the natural decline in hearing that many people experience as they get older. It is partly due to the loss of hair cells in the cochlea. It is a sensorineural hearing loss. The Rinne test, which tests air conduction vs bone conduction, is positive (normal). Although bone and air conduction are reduced equally, the relative difference between them is maintained. If air conduction is better than bone conduction (ie the normal state), the result is said to be positive. Thus, a 'positive' result indicates the healthy state, in contrast to many other medical tests.

2.23   A   Acoustic neuroma

An acoustic neuroma is a benign primary intracranial tumor of the myelin-forming cells of the vestibulocochlear nerve (CN VIII). The correct medical term is vestibular schwannoma, because it involves the vestibular portion of the 8th cranial nerve and it arises from Schwann cells, which are responsible for the myelin sheath in the peripheral nervous system. It should be suspected if there is unilateral sensorineural hearing loss and is confirmed by CT scan. The Weber test, in which a tuning fork is touched to the central forehead, localises to the normal ear in people with this condition (it does so in all cases of unilateral sensorineural deafness). Vertigo may also be a symptom.

2.24   K   Wax

Ear wax (cerumen) has cleansing, lubrication and anti-microbial roles. Excessive cerumen may impede the passage of sound in the ear canal, causing conductive hearing loss. The most common method of cerumen removal by general practitioners is syringing with warm water. It is usually necessary to soften the wax before removal, most commonly with olive oil.

2.25   H   Otosclerosis

In otosclerosis abnormal bone material grows in and around the stapes thus causing a conductive deafness. Pregnancy is not a cause but may make the condition worse, so symptoms are commonly first noticed during pregnancy. The cause is not fully understood. While it is clearly familial there is some evidence associating viral infections such as measles with otosclerosis. In many cases surgery (stapedectomy) is the treatment of choice. Diseased bone is bypassed with a prosthetic device that allows sound waves to be passed to the inner ear.

2.26   C   Chronic suppurative otitis media

Chronic suppurative otitis media is the commonest form of chronic otitis media. Clinical features are otorrhoea and conduction hearing loss of variable severity. The eardrum is perforated. It is classified into tubotympanic that is usually 'safe' and atticoantral that is often 'unsafe'. Safe or unsafe depends on the presence of cholesteatoma (a destructive and expanding sac in the middle ear). Chronic serous otitis media (otitis media with effusion) is not the same as chronic suppurative otitis media. The former may be defined as a middle ear effusion, without perforation, persisting for more than 1 to 3 months. Surgery should be considered for failure to respond to a combination of topical and systemic antibiotics. A tympanomastoidectomy can eliminate infection and stop otorrhoea in most patients. Surgery is required to remove all diseased tissue when a cholesteatoma is present.

THEME: INVESTIGATION OF LUMPS IN THE NECK

2.27   C   Excision biopsy

Unilateral parotid swelling is usually due to a pleomorphic adenoma (mixed parotid tumour). It may be indistinguishable from carcinoma clinically, although carcinoma is usually painful, rapidly growing and may cause facial nerve palsy. Excision biopsy provides diagnosis and treatment. An incomplete biopsy may seed the tumour in the wound.

2.28   B   Digital subtraction angiography

A pulsatile mass in the neck is either due to a carotid artery aneurysm or a carotid body tumour (chemodectoma). The latter is usually firm but may be soft and pulsatile. Diagnosis may be made with Doppler ultrasound or digital subtraction angiography, which is the more discriminatory test. Do not go anywhere near these masses with a needle!

2.29   D   Fine needle aspiration

A solitary thyroid nodule may be benign or malignant; secretory or non-secretory; solid or cystic; and may be 'hot' or 'cold' (depending on uptake of radio-labelled iodine). Many cold nodules are malignant but may be non-secretory adenomas. Hot nodules are usually adenomas but rarely could be follicular carcinomas. On ultrasound, cystic nodules are usually benign, solid ones may be malignant. No single radiological investigation is diagnostic. Tissue diagnosis is required for any nodule unless it is hot and cystic, or the patient is thyrotoxic. Therefore the most discriminatory test is fine needle aspiration cytology. Proceeding straight to excision biopsy will mean that many benign lesions are removed unnecessarily and that some malignant lesions are not excised completely.

2.30   K   Ultrasound

Multinodular goitre may occur in association with hyperthyroidism or, rarely, hypothyroidism. It is most commonly associated with a euthyroid state. Ultrasound will confirm the typical multinodular architecture to establish the diagnosis. Multiple nodules do not require histological investigation, as they are almost never malignant. Thyroid function tests will help guide treatment.

2.31   H   Sialogram

Salivary gland stones most commonly occur in the submandibular gland. The clinical picture as given is classic in this condition. The stone may be palpable if it is in the duct. Confirmation of the diagnosis is made with plain X-ray or contrast sialography. Stones in the duct may be expressed bimanually; stones in the gland may require surgical excision.

2.32   F   Nasopharyngoscopy

Cervical lymphadenopathy may be the first and only clinical sign of an underlying carcinoma of the pharynx, larynx, head or neck. Any lymph node that cannot be otherwise explained must be investigated with this in mind. Direct nasopharyngoscopy should be performed as a bare minimum to identify any mucosal lesions. Occasionally the diagnosis may only be made after node biopsy reveals metastatic squamous cell carcinoma but the underlying cause is usually visible when it is looked for.

2.33   A   Age related macular degeneration

Macular degeneration (AMD) is a condition predominantly of the elderly in which the macula area of the retina suffers atrophy, and in some cases, bleeding. This can result in loss of central vision. AMD begins with yellow deposits in the macula called drusen, between the retinal pigment epithelium and the underlying choroid. Most people with these early changes have good vision but can go on to develop advanced AMD. The risk is higher when the drusen are large and numerous and associated with disturbance in the pigmented cell layer under the macula. Advanced AMD has two forms: dry and wet. Central geographic atrophy, the dry form of advanced AMD, results from atrophy to the retinal pigment epithelial layer below the retina, which causes vision loss through loss of photoreceptors in the central part of the eye. Neovascular or exudative AMD, the wet form of advanced AMD, causes vision loss due to abnormal blood vessel growth in the choriocapillaries, through Bruch's membrane, ultimately leading to blood and protein leakage below the macula. Risk factors include age, family history, hypertension, high cholesterol, and obesity.

2.34   C   Posterior vitreous detachment

A posterior vitreous detachment (PVD) is a common condition in which the vitreous humour separates from the retina. Many people are not aware that they have developed PVD but some notice symptoms such as floaters or flashing lights. Floaters can take many forms from little dots, circles and lines, to clouds or cobwebs. Sometimes people experience one large floater which can be distracting and make things difficult to read. The flashing lights occur because as the outer part of the vitreous detaches from the retina it can pull on it, especially where the vitreous is attached quite strongly. The pull of the vitreous stimulates the retina. This stimulation causes the sensation of flashing lights since the brain interprets all stimulation signals from the retina as light. The only threat to vision with a posterior vitreous detachment is the small chance of a retinal tear leading to a retinal detachment.

2.35   E   Miconazole

Tinea cruris is an itchy superficial dermatophyte skin infection involving the groin and surrounding skin. As with ringworm elsewhere on the body there is a tendency for the advancing edge of the rash to be more inflamed and scaly. This is a good place to off scrape scales for laboratory examination. Microscopy is performed to look for fungal hyphae and then an attempt is made to culture the organism. Fungi such as *Trichophyton rubrum* or *Trichophyton mentagrophytes* may be isolated. If miconazole fails to clear the infection, systemic terbinafine may have to be used. Topical corticosteroids should not be applied to dermatophyte infections because they will produce tinea incognita. Corticosteroids might decrease inflammation and give a false impression that the rash is improving, while dermatophytes flourish because of immune suppression. Once the treatment is stopped the rash returns but looks different, making diagnosis difficult.

2.36   B   Malignant melanoma

Pigmented growth is seen throughout the nailbed. This is in contrast to the appearance of a subungual haematoma, which is normally associated with proximal clearing with progressive nail growth.

2.37   A   Amoxycillin

This man has acute sinusitis. It is recommended[5] that this treatment should usually be used for persistent symptoms or purulent nasal discharge lasting at least seven days or if the symptoms are severe. Doxycycline or erythromycin is an acceptable alternative. Nasal congestion can be relieved by inhalation of warm moist air or with ephedrine nasal drops.

REFERENCES

1. *Topical preparations for acne.* 13.6.1. British National Formulary; 55; 2008.

2. *Topical preparations for psoriasis.* 13.5.2. British National Formulary; 55; 2008.

3. *Topical corticosteroids.* 13.4 British National Formulary; 55; 2008.

4. S Gibbs, I Harvey, J Sterling, R Stark. Local treatments for cutaneous warts: systematic review. British Medical Journal 2002; 325, 461–464.

5. *Antibacterial drugs.* 5.1 British National Formulary; 55; 2008.

Chapter 3
Endocrinology and Metabolic

QUESTIONS

THEME: BIOCHEMISTRY OF JAUNDICE

Options

A   Dubin–Johnson syndrome
B   Extrahepatic cholestasis
C   Gilbert syndrome
D   Haemolytic jaundice
E   Intrahepatic cholestasis
F   Long-term tricyclic antidepressant use

For each of the following set of laboratory results, choose the single most likely diagnosis from the list of options above. Each option may be used once, more than once or not at all.

☐	3.1	Bilirubin 25µmol/l	Alk phos 135u/l	AST 33 IU/l	Hb 14.5g/l	No urinary bilirubin
☐	3.2	Bilirubin 85µmol/l	Alk phos 620u/l	AST 65 IU/l	Hb 14.5g/l	Bilirubin in the urine
☐	3.3	Bilirubin 58µmol/l	Alk phos 218u/l	AST 603 IU/l	Hb 14.0g/l	Bilirubin in the urine
☐	3.4	Bilirubin 35µmol/l	Alk phos 135u/l	AST 33 IU/l	Hb 10.5g/l	No urinary bilirubin

Normal values

- Bilirubin: 3–13µmol/l

- Alkaline phosphatase (Alk phos): 30–150u/l

- Aspartate transaminase (AST): 5–35 IU/l

- Haemoglobin (Hb): men 13.5–18g/l; women 11.5–16g/l

THEME: ENDOCRINE DISEASE

Options

A   Addison disease

B   Conn syndrome

C   Cushing syndrome

D   Diabetes insipidus

E   Graves' disease

F   Multiple endocrine neoplasia

G   Phaeochromocytoma

H   Syndrome of inappropriate antidiuretic hormone secretion

For each of the following clinical scenarios, choose the single most likely diagnosis from the list of options above. Each option may be used once, more than once or not at all.

☐ **3.5**   A 56-year-old woman presents to the Emergency Department with syncope. You notice she has a significant postural drop in blood pressure and also pigmentation in a recent scar on her neck.

☐ **3.6**   A 48-year-old woman has developed striae on her abdomen and is hypertensive.

☐ **3.7**   A 31-year-old woman has severe hypertension and is found to have a potassium level of 3.1mmol/l.

☐ **3.8**   A 32-year-old woman has a history of episodes of severe headache and anxiety with flushing. On examination she is very hypertensive and has a tachycardia.

THEME: HORMONAL DRUGS

Options

A   Alendronic acid

B   Bromocriptine

C   Calcitonin

D   Carbimazole

E   Cyproterone acetate

F   Desmopressin

G   Dexamethasone

H   Fludrocortisone

I   Levothyroxine sodium

J   Testosterone undecanoate

For each patient described below, choose the single most appropriate treatment from the above list of options. Each option may be used once, more than once or not at all.

☐ **3.9**   A 65-year-old woman has been taking 15mg prednisolone for 3 months to suppress bullous pemphigoid. She has a T score of -1.5 on bone mineral density scanning.

☐ **3.10**   A 50-year-old woman has tachycardia, tremor and weight loss. Her free thyroxine (T4) level is 180nmol/l.

☐ **3.11**   A 10-year-old boy with primary nocturnal enuresis wants to go on a school camping holiday.

☐ **3.12**   A 40-year-old man has Addison's disease, recently diagnosed. He attends the surgery for a repeat prescription and shows you hydrocortisone 20mg and 10mg tablets. He still feels tired and has a blood pressure of 90/50.

☐ **3.13**   An 85-year-old man has developed metastatic deposits from his prostate cancer despite treatment with the gonadorelin analogue leuprorelin acetate.

THEME: ABNORMALITIES OF WATER AND ELECTROLYTE BALANCE

Options

A Addison disease

B Conn syndrome

C Diabetes insipidus

D Renal tubular acidosis

E *Salmonella enteritis*

F Thyrotoxicosis

For each set of blood chemistry results below, choose the single most likely diagnosis from the list of options above. Each option may be used once, more than once or not at all.

☐ **3.14**	Na 136mmol/l	K 2.8mmol/l	HCO₃ 18mmol/l
☐ **3.15**	Na 149mmol/l	K 2.6mmol/l	HCO₃ 30mmol/l
☐ **3.16**	Na 128mmol/l	K 5.6mmol/l	HCO₃ 24mmol/l
☐ **3.17**	Na 130mmol/l	K 2.5mmol/l	HCO₃ 8mmol/l
☐ **3.18**	Na 160mmol/l	K 5.6mmol/l	HCO₃ 18mmol/l

Normal values

- Sodium (Na): 135–145mmol/l

- Potassium (K): 3.5–5mmol/l

- Bicarbonate (HCO₃): 24–30mmol/l

THEME: MANAGEMENT OF DIABETES MELLITUS

Options

A   Acarbose

B   Dietary modification

C   Glibenclamide

D   Gliclazide

E   Intravenous insulin sliding scale

F   Metformin

G   No change in treatment required

H   Once-daily long-acting insulin injection

I   One long-acting and three short-acting insulin injections

J   Repaglinide

K   Subcutaneous insulin sliding scale

L   Twice-daily long/short mixed insulin injections

CHAPTER 3 QUESTIONS

For each of the patients below, choose the most appropriate next management step from the list of options above. Each option may be used once, more than once or not at all.

☐ **3.19**   A 78-year-old woman is diagnosed as having diabetes after she was found to have a raised blood glucose level during an admission to hospital after a fall. Despite following appropriate dietary advice, her HbA1c remains elevated at 11%. She is not obese.

☐ **3.20**   A 27-year-old woman was found to have glycosuria at a routine antenatal clinic visit. A glucose tolerance test confirms the diagnosis of gestational diabetes.

☐ **3.21**   A 65-year-old man has had type 2 diabetes for 4 years, for which he is taking chlorpropamide. He is in hospital with an acute myocardial infarction and his laboratory blood glucose is 11mmol/l.

☐ **3.22** A 58-year-old man was diagnosed as having diabetes at a routine medical examination 3 months ago. His body mass index is 32 despite losing 5kg by following the dietician's advice. His home blood glucose readings range from 7mmol/l to 11mmol/l and his HbA1c is 10%.

☐ **3.23** A 32-year-old woman has had type 1 diabetes for 15 years. She injects isophane insulin twice a day and rarely tests her blood glucose at home. You see her for the first time in over a year and find that she is 12 weeks' pregnant.

☐ **3.24** A 65-year-old man has had type 2 diabetes for 5 years. He is on the maximum dose of tolbutamide and metformin. All his home blood glucose readings are > 11mmol/l and he complains of thirst and weight loss. His body mass index is 22.

THEME: CALCIUM AND BONE

Options

A Acromegaly
B Hyperparathyroidism
C Multiple myeloma
D Osteomalacia
E Osteoporosis
F Paget disease
G Sarcoidosis

For each of the following clinical scenarios, choose the single most likely diagnosis from the list of options above. Each option may be used once, more than once or not at all.

☐ **3.25** A 45-year-old woman presents with nausea and vomiting. She also has been experiencing some left loin pain, which is worsening.

☐ **3.26** A 51-year-old man presents with nausea, vomiting and back pain. He has recently lost some weight. He is usually very fit and active.

☐ **3.27** A 78-year-old woman presents with sudden-onset severe back pain. She is otherwise well and has no other symptoms.

☐ **3.28** A 56-year-old African Caribbean patient present with nausea and vomiting associated with increased shortness of breath. He is usually very fit and well and is not taking any medications. He is also complaining of sore eyes.

3.29   A 23-year-old insulin dependent patient comes to your clinic for pre-pregnancy counselling with regard to her glycaemic control and the right time to try for a baby.

Which one of the following options is the best test that will help you advise the patient?

- ☐ **A**   HbA1c
- ☐ **B**   1-hour glucose tolerance test (GTT)
- ☐ **C**   2-hour GTT
- ☐ **D**   Random blood sugar
- ☐ **E**   Sugar series

3.30   A 50-year-old woman has a 2 hour glucose level of 9.0mmol/l on the 75g oral glucose tolerance test. Her body mass index is 33.

Select from the list below the single most likely diagnosis.

- ☐ **A**   Impaired fasting glucose
- ☐ **B**   Impaired glucose tolerance
- ☐ **C**   Normal level
- ☐ **D**   Type 1 diabetes mellitus
- ☐ **E**   Type 2 diabetes mellitus

3.31   **Select from the list below the single false statement relating to the assessment of obesity in an adult.**

☐   **A**   Body mass index (BMI) between 18.5 and 24.9 signifies a healthy weight

☐   **B**   BMI may not be an accurate guide in highly muscular people

☐   **C**   In the classification of obesity, severe obesity (obesity III) is recognised with a BMI > 40

☐   **D**   The decision on management is made independently of the presence of any co-morbidity

☐   **E**   Waist circumference is a useful adjunct in assessing patients with lower levels of obesity (overweight and obesity I)

3.32   **A frail 85-year-old woman has evidence of a compression fracture of a thoracic vertebra. You are considering treatment with a bisphosphonate.**

        Select from the list below the single true statement.

☐   **A**   A bone mineral density (BMD) T score of between 0 and -1 is required before starting the bisphosphonate

☐   **B**   A T score of between -1 and -2.5 is needed

☐   **C**   A T score below -2.5 is needed

☐   **D**   Calcium (0.5–1g) and vitamin D (800 IU) alone is the correct treatment

☐   **E**   None of these is true

CHAPTER 3 QUESTIONS

3.33 A 66-year-old obese man is brought into the Emergency Department semiconscious. His cleaner found him unwell in bed. He takes bendroflumethiazide for his hypertension. It is known that he had had diarrhoea and vomiting two days ago. His biochemistry profile is:

Na 154mmol/l	K 5.9mmol/l	Urea 21.0mmol/l	Cr 160μmol/l	Gluc 45mmol/l

Normal values

- Sodium (Na): 135–145mmol/l

- Potassium (K): 3.5–5mmol/l

- Urea (Ur): 2.5–6.7mmol/l

- Creatinine (Cr): 70 < 150μmol/l

- Glucose fasting: 3.5–6.0mmol/l

From the list below select the single most appropriate diagnosis.

☐ **A** Acute renal failure
☐ **B** Dehydration
☐ **C** Diabetic ketoacidosis
☐ **D** Drug toxicity
☐ **E** Hyperosmolar non-ketotic coma

ANSWERS

THEME: BIOCHEMISTRY OF JAUNDICE

3.1   C   Gilbert syndrome

In Gilbert syndrome the bilirubin is unconjugated due to congenital failure of the hepatocytes to take up the bilirubin for conjugation. Therefore there is no bilirubin in the urine as only the conjugated form is water soluble and appears in the urine. Dubin–Johnson syndrome is the congenital failure of excretion of the conjugated bilirubin into the bile canaliculi.

3.2   B   Extrahepatic cholestasis

The very elevated alkaline phosphatase in the presence of jaundice indicates extrahepatic obstruction, typically from a common bile duct stone or carcinoma of the head of the pancreas.

3.3   E   Intrahepatic cholestasis

In intrahepatic cholestasis, the AST is very elevated but the alkaline phosphatase, which arises from the bile duct walls, is not. Common causes are drugs, alcohol and infective hepatitis.

3.4   D   Haemolytic jaundice

In haemolytic jaundice there will be anaemia. There is no elevation in urinary bilirubin because the haemolysis releases unconjugated bilirubin, which is not water soluble and therefore will not appear in the urine.

THEME: ENDOCRINE DISEASE

3.5   A   Addison disease

Primary hypoadrenalism due to destruction of the adrenal cortex leads to a reduction in glucocorticoid, mineralocorticoid and sex steroid production. Reduced cortisol levels produce an increase in adrenocorticotropic hormone (ACTH) production by the pituitary, which is responsible for the pigmentation by its action on melanocytes. Postural hypotension is due to hypovolaemia and sodium loss.

3.6   C   Cushing syndrome

Cushing syndrome is due to an increase in the secretion of glucocorticoids. In Cushing disease there is an increase in ACTH production by the pituitary gland. Other causes are ACTH-producing tumours and non-ACTH dependent causes such as an adrenal adenoma.

3.7   B   Conn syndrome

Primary hyperaldosteronism causes sodium retention, hypertension and hypokalaemia. Conn syndrome is due to an adrenal adenoma, but adrenal hyperplasia can also cause the condition.

3.8   G   Phaeochromocytoma

Tumours that release noradrenaline and adrenaline (norepinephrine and epinephrine) frequently cause intermittent symptoms. Most phaeochromocytomas arise from the adrenal glands. Some are associated with the multiple endocrine neoplasia syndromes.

THEME: HORMONAL DRUGS

3.9   A   Alendronic acid

Current guidelines[1] suggest that, at this level of T score, treatment should be considered for glucocorticoid induced osteoporosis. The bisphosphonate alendronic acid 5mg daily would normally be the drug of first choice. Calcium and vitamin D would usually be given as adjuncts. Intranasal calcitonin is licensed for the treatment of postmenopausal osteoporosis but the data is inconsistent for glucocorticoid induced bone loss.

3.10   D   Carbimazole

Antithyroid drugs are used for hyperthyroidism, either to prepare patients for thyroidectomy or for long term management. Carbimazole is the drug most commonly given in the UK. The dose is usually 15–40mg daily and is reduced when the patient becomes euthyroid. An alternative is the blocking-replacement regimen when a larger dose (40–60mg) daily is given in combination with levothyroxine for about 18 months. Carbimazole can cause neutropenia and agranulocytosis and patients should be warned to report infections, especially sore throat.

3.11   F   Desmopressin

Desmopressin is an analogue of vasopressin (antidiuretic hormone). It can be taken by mouth, sublingually or as a nasal spray to treat primary nocturnal enuresis. Patients are cautioned to limit fluid intake to a minimum for one hour before dose until 8 hours after to minimise the risk of hyponatraemic convulsions. Similarly the drug should be stopped during episodes of vomiting and diarrhoea. Many doctors would prescribe the drug for a short period to cover something like a school camping holiday.

3.12   H   Fludrocortisone

In Addison disease hydrocortisone is given as replacement therapy usually in two doses, the larger in the morning to mimic the diurnal rhythm of cortisol secretion. Hydrocortisone only has weak mineralocorticoid activity so fludrocortisone needs to be given as well to ensure complete replacement of absent hormones. There seems to have been some failure of communication here between hospital and patient.

3.13   E   Cyproterone acetate

Treatment of metastatic prostate cancer is usually aimed at depleting androgen either by orchidectomy or by using a gonadorelin analogue. The latter initially causes a stimulation of the pituitary and later a decrease of luteinising hormone release. The consequent initial rise in testosterone may lead to a tumour 'flare' in susceptible individuals. The anti-androgen drug cyproterone acetate can be used to control this 'flare' for the first 2–3 weeks of treatment with the gonadorelin analogue. It can also be used alone when treatment with the latter drug has failed. It is also used in dermatology in a combination with ethinylestradiol to treat acne and hirsuitism.

THEME: ABNORMALITIES OF WATER AND ELECTROLYTE BALANCE

3.14   D   Renal tubular acidosis

The hallmark of renal tubular acidosis is a mild metabolic acidosis with hypokalaemia. The normal range for serum bicarbonate concentration is 24–30mmol/l. The low level suggests acidosis. The clinical picture is common after treatment with acetazolamide.

3.15   B   Conn syndrome

Conn syndrome or primary hyperaldosteronism is a rare condition, but it is important as a cause of secondary arterial hypertension. The main clinical feature is hypertension without oedema and the combination of mild hypernatraemia with hypokalaemia.

3.16   A   Addison disease

Addison disease or adrenal failure is characterised by low blood pressure, pigmentation of the skin and buccal mucosa, and the combination of hyponatraemia and mild hyperkalaemia.

3.17   E   *Salmonella enteritis*

Severe diarrhoea results in metabolic acidosis due to bicarbonate loss and hypokalaemia. (Remember: the bicarbonate content of bowel is approximately 80mmol/l.)

3.18   C   Diabetes insipidus

Diabetes insipidus is due to antidiuretic hormone (ADH) deficiency or lack/loss of renal ADH responsiveness. These patients lose predominantly free water and present with polyuria and dehydration. Other causes of a similar electrolyte pattern are poor fluid intake or water loss due to fever/hyperventilation.

THEME: MANAGEMENT OF DIABETES MELLITUS

3.19   D   Gliclazide

This patient will almost certainly have type 2 diabetes. Diet alone will control the diabetes for many of these patients. If that does not happen, the patient requires an oral hypoglycaemic agent. Biguanides (metformin) are the drugs of choice if the patient is obese unless they have cardiac or renal failure. Sulphonylureas are the drugs of choice if the patient is not obese. In older patients, a short-acting agent minimises the risk of hypoglycaemia or drug accumulation if there is impairment of renal function. Glibenclamide and chlorpropamide are longest acting and, therefore, least safe. Gliclazide and tolbutamide are shorter acting and safer.

CHAPTER 3 ANSWERS

3.20   B   Dietary modification

Gestational diabetes (diabetes arising for the first time in pregnancy) is often treatable with diet control alone. The patient needs to be counselled well and must be encouraged to monitor blood glucose at home. A few women will require insulin to achieve glycaemic control. Oral hypoglycaemics should not be used in pregnancy. Glycosuria is common in pregnancy due to lowering of the renal threshold. If glycosuria is persistently present, a glucose tolerance test should be done. Some women with gestational diabetes either remain diabetic or subsequently develop diabetes.

3.21   E   Intravenous insulin sliding scale

There is good evidence that cardiac mortality is reduced with the use of insulin following myocardial infarction. Any patient with a known diagnosis of diabetes, regardless of treatment, or with a blood glucose >8.0mmol/l at presentation with an acute myocardial infarction should receive insulin treatment. The regimen used in the landmark trial was 3 days on an intravenous insulin sliding scale followed by 3 months on subcutaneous insulin. The subgroup of patients converted to insulin from sulphonylureas benefited the most.[2]

3.22   F   Metformin

This man's type 2 diabetes is inadequately controlled (preprandial blood glucose should be 4–7mmol/l and HbA1c should be < 7.0%). Metformin is the drug of choice, as he is obese. If this fails, acarbose or a sulphonylurea may be tried.

3.23   I   One long-acting and three short-acting insulin injections

Pregnant women with diabetes have an increased risk of most maternal and fetal complications, and an increased risk of accelerated complication of diabetes. Particular risks are intrauterine death, premature labour, pre-eclampsia, congenital malformations and neonatal mortality. There is good evidence that tight glycaemic control improves outcome but at the expense of increasing the mother's risk of hypoglycaemia. A four times daily regimen (three injections of soluble insulin and one injection of long-acting insulin) has recently been shown to reduce the risk of hypoglycaemic attacks. The patient in this question will require considerable support and counselling.

3.24   H   Once-daily long-acting insulin injection

A patient with type 2 diabetes may require insulin if good glycaemic control cannot be achieved with diet and oral medication. If a patient is on metformin and a sulphonylurea and is obese, then acarbose or repaglinide may be tried. If they are not obese, insulin is required. Insulin may be given instead of oral medication. It is more usual to add a once-daily dose of long-acting insulin to the oral regimen. This patient is symptomatic so should probably receive insulin even if he were obese.

THEME: CALCIUM AND BONE

3.25   B   Hyperparathyroidism

Primary hyperparathyroidism is usually due to a single parathyroid adenoma. It may cause renal calculi. Treatment is by surgical excision of the underlying parathyroid tumour(s).

3.26   C   Multiple myeloma

This patient's symptoms of hypercalcaemia are due to excessive bone destruction. Bone pain, particularly back pain, is the commonest symptom of myeloma and is caused by vertebral collapse and nerve entrapment. Myeloma is diagnosed by the presence of a monoclonal protein, usually IgG or IgA, in the serum in 80% of cases. In the remainder, light chains (Bence Jones protein) can be detected in the urine.

3.27   E   Osteoporosis

A wedge fracture due to osteoporosis is the most likely diagnosis in this woman as she is otherwise asymptomatic. Many people with osteoporosis are unaware they have it until they present with a facture.

3.28   G   Sarcoidosis

Sarcoidosis is a systemic disease with non-caseating granuloma in lymph nodes and other sites. It is a recognised cause of hypercalcaemia and is more common in people of African Caribbean origin. It can be associated with anterior and posterior uveitis. Treatment is usually with corticosteroids.

3.29   A   HbA1c

This best measures the average blood glucose concentration over the lifespan of a haemoglobin molecule, which is approximately 6 weeks. Levels below 6% are considered to be a reflection of good glycaemic control and the patient can start trying for a baby at this stage. Folic acid supplementation is necessary as a preventative measure because diabetic mothers have an increased risk of having babies with neural tube defects.

3.30   B   Impaired glucose tolerance

A patient is said to have impaired glucose tolerance (IGT) when she has an intermediately raised glucose level after 2 hours, but less than would signify type 2 diabetes mellitus (> 11mmol/l). The fasting glucose may be either normal or mildly elevated. An elevated fasting glucose level of 6.1–6.9mmol/l signifies impaired fasting glucose (IFG). Patients with IGT or IFG are at increased risk of developing type II diabetes and cardiovascular morbidity. They often have other features of the metabolic syndrome: obesity, dyslipidaemia and hypertension. Management involves dietary modification and risk factor management to attempt to prevent progression.

3.31   D   The decision on management is made independently of the presence of any co-morbidity

NICE[3] includes recommendations on classification (Table 1) and assessment (Table 2) in its guidelines on the management of overweight and obesity in adults.

Table 1: Classifying overweight and obesity

Classification	BMI (kg/m^2)
Healthy weight	18.5–24.9
Overweight	25–29.9
Obesity I	30–34.9
Obesity II	35–39.9
Obesity III	> 40

CHAPTER 3 ANSWERS

Table 2: Assessing risks from overweight and obesity

BMI CLASSIFICATION	WAIST CIRCUMFERENCE*		
	LOW	HIGH	VERY HIGH
Overweight	No increased risk	Increased risk	High risk
Obesity I	Increased risk	High risk	Very high risk

*For men, waist circumference of < 94cm is low, 94–102cm is high and > 102cm is very high

*For women, waist circumference of < 80cm is low, 80–88cm is high and > 88cm is very high.

Management consists of diet and physical activity and for patients with obesity II a consideration of drugs and for obesity III surgery. The presence of co-morbidity lowers the threshold for considering drugs and surgery. Co-morbidities include type 2 diabetes, hypertension, cardiovascular disease, dyslipidaemia, osteoarthritis and sleep apnoea.

3.32   E   None of these is true

A bone mineral density (BMD) T score of zero is regarded as average peak bone mass and between 0 and -1 is normal; -1 to -2.5 is osteopenia and in the absence of a previous fracture requires only lifestyle advice. Below -2.5 is osteoporosis and a bisphosphonate or other suitable treatment is indicated. For patients taking glucocorticoids the corresponding figure is -1.5. Calcium and vitamin D are generally regarded as adjuncts to treatment. They should be given anyway to any frail patient who has an increased risk of falls. A previous fragility fracture (as in this patient) is a strong independent risk for further fracture and may be regarded as an indication for treatment without the need for BMD measurement.[4]

3.33   E   Hyperosmolar non-ketotic coma

This is a condition that signifies a type 2 diabetic (non-insulin-dependent diabetes mellitus, NIDDM) emergency. Severe hyperglycaemia leads to profound dehydration and patients develop a hyperosmolar state (osmolality = 2([Na+] + [K+]) + [Glu] + [Urea]). However, there is no ketosis in contrast to the diabetic emergency of ketoacidosis seen in type 1 diabetics. Due to the hyperosmolar state, patients often have a decreased level of consciousness on presentation.

REFERENCES

1. Bone and Tooth Society of Great Britain, National Osteoporosis Society, Royal College of Physicians. *Glucocorticoid-induced osteoporosis: Guidelines on prevention and treatment.* December 2002.

2. Malmberg K, Ryden L, Hamsten A , Herlitz J, Waldenström A, Wedel H, Welin L. Randomized trial of insulin-glucose infusion followed by subcutaneous insulin treatment in diabetic patients with acute myocardial infarction (DIGAMI study); effects on mortality at 1 year. J Am Coll Cardiol 26:56–65, 1995.

3. National Institute for Health and Clinical Excellence. *Obesity: Guidance on the prevention, identification, assessment and management of overweight and obesity in adults and children. Quick Reference Guide* (homepage on the Internet), December 2006 (cited 2008 April 23). Available from http://www.nice.org.uk/nicemedia/pdf/CG43quickrefguide2.pdf

4. Royal College of Physicians and Bone and Tooth Society of Great Britain. Osteoporosis – clinical guidelines for prevention and treatment. *Update on pharmacological interventions and an algorithm for management.* July 2000.

CHAPTER 3 ANSWERS

Chapter 4
Gastroenterology and Nutrition

QUESTIONS

THEME: CAUSES OF CONSTIPATION

Options

A   Anal fissure

B   Bed rest

C   Bowel obstruction

D   Carcinoma of the colon

E   Carcinoma of the rectum

F   Depression

G   Hypercalcaemia

H   Hypothyroidism

I   Iatrogenic

J   Irritable bowel syndrome

K   Poor fibre intake

L   Pregnancy

For each of the patients below, choose the single most likely diagnosis from the list of options above. Each option may be used once, more than once or not at all.

☐ **4.1**   A 60-year-old woman presents with a 3-day history of constipation, colicky abdominal pain, distension and vomiting. She has not even passed wind. Bowel sounds are active and high pitched.

☐ **4.2**   A 30-year-old man complains of constipation and pain on defaecation. He also notices small amounts of fresh blood on the paper afterwards. He is unable to tolerate a rectal examination.

☐ **4.3**   A 21-year-old woman with mild learning difficulties complains of recent onset of abdominal distension, constipation, indigestion and amenorrhoea.

☐ **4.4**   A 65-year-old man complains of constipation, low mood, low back pain that prevents him sleeping, fatigue and thirst. He has bony tenderness over his lumbar spine.

☐ **4.5**   A 52-year-old woman complains of constipation and nausea 4 days after abdominal hysterectomy for fibroids. On examination she has active bowel sounds of normal pitch and pinpoint pupils.

☐ **4.6**   A 60-year-old man presents with a 2-month history of increasing constipation with occasional diarrhoea. He also describes anorexia, weight loss and a feeling of tenesmus.

THEME: CAUSES OF HEPATOMEGALY

Options

A Acute myeloid leukaemia

B Amyloidosis

C Congestive cardiac failure

D Chronic lymphocytic leukaemia

E Chronic myeloid leukaemia

F Hepatocellular carcinoma

G Infectious mononucleosis

H Liver metastases

I Lymphoma

J Malaria

K Myelofibrosis

L Tricuspid regurgitation

For each of the patients below, choose the single most likely diagnosis from the list of options above. Each option may be used once, more than once or not at all.

☐ **4.7** A 20-year-old student presents to her GP with a 1-week history of fever and sore throat. On examination, she has tender cervical lymphadenopathy and an enlarged, tender liver.

☐ **4.8** A 62-year-old man presents with a 3-month history of intermittent constipation and diarrhoea and progressive weight loss. On examination, he is cachectic and has knobbly hepatomegaly. He is not jaundiced. His liver function is normal.

☐ **4.9** An 81-year-old woman presents with a 6-month history of abdominal swelling, hepatomegaly and leg oedema. She has a history of rheumatic fever as a child and hypertension for the past few years. She takes atenolol for her hypertension.

☐ **4.10** A 56-year-old woman has a 20-year history of rheumatoid arthritis. Despite numerous drugs, her arthritis has only recently been under control. Recently she has noticed that she bruises easily. On examination she has a large beefy tongue, lymphadenopathy and hepatomegaly.

☐ **4.11** A 31-year-old man presents to casualty with a 2-week history of night sweats, weight loss and pruritus. He has noticed some enlarged glands in his groin that become painful if he drinks alcohol. On examination he has no other evidence of lymphadenopathy but there is a smooth enlarged liver.

THEME: CAUSES OF DYSPHAGIA

Options

A   Achalasia

B   Bronchial carcinoma

C   Carcinoma of the oesophagus

D   Chronic benign stricture

E   Left atrial hypertrophy

F   Myasthenia gravis

G   Oesophageal candidosis

H   Pharyngeal pouch

I   Plummer–Vinson syndrome

J   Reflux oesophagitis

K   Thoracic aneurysm

For each of the patients below, choose the most likely diagnosis from the list of options above. Each option may be used once, more than once or not at all.

☐ **4.12**   A 50-year-old obese woman complains of a burning retrosternal discomfort after eating and on lying down. She has also noticed excessive salivation and wheezing when she lies down to sleep.

☐ **4.13**   A 35-year-old housewife has noticed progressively worsening difficulty swallowing over several years. She has been troubled by regurgitation of undigested food and halitosis, and has fits of coughing on lying flat.

☐ **4.14**   A 45-year-old pale woman complains that food is sticking in the back of her throat. On examination she has spoon-shaped nails, a smooth tongue and angular cheilitis.

☐ **4.15** A 75-year-old man complains of difficulty in swallowing. He finds that the first mouthful of food is easy to swallow but thereafter he has increasing difficulty in swallowing until he regurgitates undigested food. He also notices a neck swelling.

☐ **4.16** A 60-year-old woman complains of difficulty swallowing. On examination she has a prominent malar flush, an irregularly irregular pulse and raised jugular venous pressure. On auscultation there is a rumbling, long, low-pitched, mid-diastolic murmur best heard in the left lateral position in expiration.

THEME: ACUTE ABDOMEN

Options

A   Acute salpingitis

B   Adhesive small bowel obstruction

C   Appendicitis

D   Leaking aortic aneurysm

E   Mesenteric ischaemia

F   Pancreatitis

G   Perforated peptic ulcer

H   Torsion of an ovarian cyst

I   Ureteric colic

For each of the patients below, choose the single most likely diagnosis from the list of options above. Each option may be used once, more than once or not at all.

☐ **4.17**   A 60-year-old man with epigastric pain and brief collapse at home is now alert with some mild back pain and tachycardia.

☐ **4.18**   A 45-year-old man has been taking ibuprofen for persistent abdominal pain. He has been brought to the Emergency Department after a sudden collapse, and an erect chest film shows gas under the diaphragm.

☐ **4.19**   A 36-year-old woman has been brought to the Emergency Department by her husband with very severe left-sided abdominal pain. Her husband states that she has been pacing around the bedroom all night, unable to find a comfortable position, and the patient describes the pain as being 'worse than a labour pain'.

☐ **4.20** An 87-year-old woman is admitted with a rigid abdomen. A careful history reveals she has been having pain after meals and has stopped eating very much. Her blood gas assay reveals a metabolic acidosis. Her amylase level is within normal limits.

☐ **4.21** A 23-year-old woman presents with right iliac fossa pain for 4 days, associated with nausea but no vomiting. A dipstick urine test is normal and a careful history reveals offensive vaginal discharge.

THEME: UPPER ABDOMINAL PAIN

Options

A	Bleeding peptic ulcer	**F**	Myocardial infarction
B	Biliary colic	**G**	Pancreatitis
C	Cholecystitis	**H**	Perforated peptic ulcer
D	Gastric outlet obstruction	**I**	Ulcerative colitis
E	Lower lobe pneumonia		

For each of the scenarios described below, select the single most likely diagnosis from the list of options above. Each option may be used once, more than once or not at all.

☐ **4.22** A 33-year-old woman presents with severe abdominal pain radiating to the back. She is shocked and hyperventilating. There is no free gas on her erect chest X-ray. A right-sided opacity is noted at the level of the L1 vertebra.

☐ **4.23** A 57-year-old smoker presents with epigastric pain, and sweating, and is vomiting clear fluid. He has a pulse of 58 and a raised jugular venous pressure.

☐ **4.24** A 43-year-old man with multiple sclerosis presents with a pulse of 120 and a rigid abdomen. He is apyrexial. There are no bowel sounds. He has recently completed a course of methylprednisolone.

☐ **4.25** A 47-year-old woman presents with intermittent epigastric pain and vomiting. The pain can last for hours. She has mild epigastric and right upper quadrant tenderness. Bowel sounds are present.

☐ **4.26** An 83-year-old man presents following a collapse. He is not tachycardic but has a postural drop in blood pressure. He has mild epigastric discomfort. You note he has a history of arthritis and hypertension and takes diclofenac and atenolol for these conditions.

THEME: MANAGEMENT OF CONSTIPATION

Options

A Isphaghula husk

B Lactulose

C Lidocaine hydrochloride

D Loperamide

E Macrogol (polyethylene glycol)

F Mebeverine hydrochloride

G Senna

H Sodium acid phosphate

For each of the scenarios below select the single most appropriate medication from the above list. Each option may be used once, more than once or not at all.

☐ **4.27**   A 55-year-old woman has been investigated for constipation and told she has diverticulosis. She remains relatively constipated and intermittently needs stimulant laxatives. Her diet seems adequate.

☐ **4.28**   A 40-year-old man has had acute low back pain for one week. He has obtained pain relief using a combination of paracetamol and codeine but constipation has become a problem.

☐ **4.29**   An 80-year-old man has ischaemic heart disease and osteoarthritis for which he takes a large number of drugs. He has long standing constipation and takes an osmotic laxative and a stimulant laxative. He has taken to his bed because of a flu-like illness. He is now unable to pass a stool, has a very uncomfortable feeling of fullness in the rectum and is leaking watery faecal material from his anus.

☐ **4.30**   A 35-year-old man finds it very painful to pass a stool and has been trying to suppress the urge and consequently has become constipated. He has noticed blood on the toilet paper when he wipes himself.

4.31   A 56-year-old-man, who attends surgery infrequently, presents with a 5-week history of heartburn and acid reflux. He returns to see you after a 2-week trial of a proton pump inhibitor (PPI) with partial improvement. His body mass index is 25.

Which one of the following is the most appropriate next step in his management?

☐ **A**   Add an alginate preparation

☐ **B**   Continue the PPI and review in 2 weeks

☐ **C**   *Helicobacter pylori* testing

☐ **D**   Refer for urgent endoscopy

☐ **E**   Refer to a dietician for advice including weight loss measures

4.32   Regarding irritable bowel syndrome, which one of the following statements is correct?

☐ **A**   It is a cause of rectal bleeding

☐ **B**   It is more prevalent in women

☐ **C**   It often has oral symptoms

☐ **D**   It usually presents in childhood

☐ **E**   Weight loss is common

CHAPTER 4 QUESTIONS

4.33 A 45-year-old man has suffered recurrent episodes of epigastric pain for several years. His symptoms responded to proton pump inhibitor (PPI) but relapsed after stopping. A test for *Helicobacter pylori* was positive but after initial improvement after eradication therapy the symptoms relapsed.

Select from the list below the single most appropriate next step in management.

- [ ] **A** Add an alginate preparation
- [ ] **B** Prescribe a PPI again
- [ ] **C** Refer for urgent endoscopy
- [ ] **D** Refer to a dietician for advice including weight loss measures
- [ ] **E** Retest for *H. pylori*

4.34 A 30-year-old woman has general lassitude and persistent loose stools. She was found to be iron deficient but response to treatment has been slow. You suspect she may have coeliac disease.

Select from the list below the single most appropriate initial investigation.

- [ ] **A** Endomysium antibody (EMA)
- [ ] **B** Endomysium antibody plus IgA level
- [ ] **C** Gluten challenge
- [ ] **D** Jejunal biopsy
- [ ] **E** 24-hour faecal fat

4.35   A 40-year-old woman has intermittent central abdominal pain and bloating. Sometimes she is constipated; sometimes her stools are loose and sometimes normal. She often feels better after passing a stool. Nothing abnormal is found on investigation.

Select from the list below the single most appropriate investigation that should be carried out.

- [ ] **A**   Abdominal ultrasound
- [ ] **B**   Barium enema
- [ ] **C**   Colonoscopy
- [ ] **D**   Plain X-ray abdomen
- [ ] **E**   None of these

ANSWERS

THEME: CAUSES OF CONSTIPATION

4.1   C   Bowel obstruction

Absolute constipation (ie inability to pass flatus as well as faeces) is one of the cardinal features of bowel obstruction. The other features are colicky abdominal pain, distension and vomiting. In small-bowel obstruction, constipation appears after the onset of vomiting; in large-bowel obstruction, vomiting appears later. High-pitched bowel sounds are strongly suggestive of mechanical bowel obstruction. Functional obstruction (pseudo-obstruction) may cause a similar clinical picture but the bowel sounds are often absent.

4.2   A   Anal fissure

Anal fissure is a very common problem and often follows a period of relative constipation. The passage of a hard stool produces a fissure, the pain of which causes anal spasm and further constipation. The resultant vicious cycle can be broken with stool softeners and local anaesthetic preparations. Topical nitrates have also proved useful in reducing spasm. Severe cases may require an anal stretch or lateral sphincterotomy under anaesthesia.

4.3   L   Pregnancy

Pregnancy causes constipation due to the presence of a pelvic mass and reduced gastrointestinal motility. Indigestion occurs later as smooth muscle relaxation reduces the tone of the gastro-oesophageal sphincter and results in acid reflux. Pregnancy in young women may present late, even in the absence of learning difficulties.

4.4   G   Hypercalcaemia

The combination of depression, fatigue, constipation and bone pain is suggestive of hypercalcaemia. In a man of this age, the likely cause is malignant disease. Back pain that prevents the patient sleeping is also suspicious for metastases or myeloma. Hypothyroidism could also explain most of the symptoms but not the back pain. Colorectal carcinoma does not usually produce bone metastases.

4.5   I   Iatrogenic

Patients in hospital often develop constipation for a number of reasons including pain, poor fluid intake, lack of dietary fibre, immobility and medication. It would be unlikely that a routine hysterectomy would result in bowel obstruction directly. However, it is likely that opioid analgesia, given for postoperative pain, will cause constipation if adequate fluids, fibre and/or laxatives are not provided. Nausea may be due to impending bowel obstruction or due directly to the opioids. Pinpoint pupils also suggest the patient is receiving excess opioids.

4.6   E   Carcinoma of the rectum

Tenesmus, the feeling that the bowel is incompletely emptied after evacuation, is a symptom that is associated with rectal tumours (carcinoma or polyps) and irritable bowel syndrome. It is unusual for irritable bowel syndrome to develop in a patient of older age and the presence of anorexia and weight loss is more consistent with cancer.

THEME: CAUSES OF HEPATOMEGALY

4.7   G   Infectious mononucleosis

Glandular fever (infectious mononucleosis) may cause liver or spleen enlargement in about 10% of cases. Occasionally the organs are painful due to rapid expansion causing stretching of the capsule. Rarely, splenic enlargement may be so rapid that the spleen is liable to rupture. Liver function tests are often abnormal but rarely done.

4.8   H   Liver metastases

Liver metastases commonly arise from bowel and breast. Palpable metastases need not have any effect on liver function, which is only impaired if the metastases involve over half the liver or if there is biliary obstruction.

4.9   C   Congestive cardiac failure

Right heart failure is often forgotten as a cause of ascites and hepatomegaly, due to congestive changes. In tricuspid regurgitation, the enlarged liver may be pulsatile. The commonest causes of right heart failure are left heart failure, hypertension and valvular disease. Rheumatic fever rarely causes tricuspid or pulmonary valve lesions, so this patient probably has cardiac failure primarily due to aortic or mitral valve disease or hypertension.

CHAPTER 4 ANSWERS

4.10   B   Amyloidosis

Patients with chronic inflammatory diseases may develop secondary amyloidosis. Causative conditions include rheumatoid arthritis, bronchiectasis and chronic osteomyelitis. Amyloid accumulates in lymphoreticular and other tissues, such as the tongue and skin. Purpura may be due to cutaneous amyloid or hypersplenism-induced thrombocytopenia. Cardiac amyloid is rare in secondary amyloid. Amyloid also causes nephrotic syndrome. Felty syndrome is the main differential diagnosis in a patient with hepatosplenomegaly and rheumatoid arthritis. However, in this syndrome patients also have lymphadenopathy, neutropenia, anaemia and thrombocytopenia. The main complication is infection.

4.11   I   Lymphoma

Patients with lymphoma may either present with a lump (or lumps) or with generalised symptoms. Of particular importance are 'B symptoms' – weight loss, fever, night sweats – which affect the choice of treatment and prognosis of the disease. Involvement of extra-nodal sites, such as liver, spleen and bone marrow, puts this patient at stage 4B. This is the highest stage and carries the worst prognosis. Treatment is chemotherapy after histological confirmation. Lymph node pain on drinking alcohol is said to be a feature of Hodgkins disease.

THEME: CAUSES OF DYSPHAGIA

4.12   J   Reflux oesophagitis

Gastro-oesophageal reflux disease (GORD) is associated with smoking, high alcohol intake, hiatus hernia, pregnancy, obesity, systemic sclerosis and tight clothes. Gastric acid enters the oesophagus through the incompetent lower oesophageal sphincter. This results in oesophageal inflammation, which if extensive may result in dysphagia and eventually oesophageal stricture or Barrett's oesophagus. (The normal stratified squamous epithelium of the distal oesophagus is replaced by an abnormal columnar epithelium that pridisposes to malignancy.) Patients may complain of heartburn, an acid taste in the mouth (acid brash), excessive salivation (waterbrash), difficulty in swallowing and nocturnal asthma.

4.13   A   Achalasia

Oesophageal achalasia involves failure of relaxation of the circular muscles at the lower end of the oesophagus associated with loss of the myenteric plexus of nerves in this region. Oesophageal dilatation occurs above the area of achalasia. The condition tends to present between the ages of 30 and 40 years and is slightly more common in women. Dysphagia gradually progresses over years. In addition to regurgitation of partially digested food and halitosis, patients may aspirate on lying flat (hence the coughing) and so are susceptible to aspiration pneumonia. The diagnosis may be obvious on a chest X-ray showing a wide mediastinum and a shadow behind the heart with a fluid level. The diagnosis can be confirmed with a barium swallow or endoscopy. Treatment of severe achalasia is usually surgical (Heller operation – longitudinal division of the lowest part of the oesophagal muscle) but mild achalasia may respond to nitrates and anticholinergic medication.

4.14   I   Plummer–Vinson syndrome

Plummer–Vinson syndrome or Paterson–Brown–Kelly syndrome consists of iron deficiency anaemia, glossitis, angular cheilitis and dysphagia due to a postcricoid oesophageal web. A friable web lies across the anterior oesophageal lumen and may be seen on endoscopy and a barium meal. It is caused by epithelial hyperplasia and hyperkeratosis of the oesophageal mucosa. The condition is premalignant and the patient should undergo biopsy. The iron deficiency anaemia should be investigated and treated appropriately.

4.15   H   Pharyngeal pouch

The development of a pharyngeal pouch is often preceded by a history suggestive of reflux oesophagitis or hiatus hernia. It has been hypothesised that oesophageal hypertrophy occurs in an attempt to prevent acid reflux and that this causes a relative obstruction at the level of cricopharyngeus muscle with the resultant pressure causing protrusion of a mucosal pouch at the level of Killian dehiscence between thyreopharyngeus and cricopharyngeus. This pouch is usually easily demonstrated in the upper neck on a barium swallow. Again patients are prone to aspiration of semi-digested food which leads to episodes of coughing and aspiration pneumonia. Management is surgical with excision of the pouch.

4.16   E   Left atrial hypertrophy

The description of the clinical findings suggests that this patient has significant mitral stenosis. The associated large left atrium may favour atrial fibrillation with palpitations and pressure on the oesophagus may result in dysphagia. Radiological features of mitral stenosis associated with enlargement of the left atrium include a double cardiac silhouette, straightening of the left border of the heart and a horizontal left bronchus.

THEME: ACUTE ABDOMEN

4.17   D   Leaking aortic aneurysm

A leaking abdominal aortic aneurysm may mimic many other causes of acute abdomen. The classic triad of a pulsatile mass, severe back pain and profound hypotensive collapse has a poor prognosis, and these patients frequently do not make it to hospital alive. The clues here are the age, the sex and the signs of cardiovascular instability.

4.18 G Perforated peptic ulcer

Non-steroidal anti-inflammatory drugs are widely used, and have a detrimental effect on the kidneys and the gastrointestinal tract. Gas under the diaphragm indicates a perforated viscus and these patients will usually have advanced signs of peritonitis.

4.19 I Ureteric colic

The pain of ureteric colic is very severe and will often be described as the worst pain a patient has ever experienced. The characteristic restlessness and inability to find a position that is comfortable is highly suggestive of this condition. A dipstick urine test will usually be positive for blood, and a ureteric calculus will sometimes be seen on X-ray.

4.20 E Mesenteric ischaemia

Mesenteric ischaemia occurs in patients with arteriopathy. Risk factors therefore include an arrhythmia such as atrial fibrillation, advanced age, smoking and diabetes. Postprandial pain and weight loss may denote so-called 'mesenteric angina'. Progression to intestinal gangrene may show as dilated loops of bowel with 'thumb printing' on a plain abdominal X-ray film, and a blood gas assay may show a metabolic acidosis with profound base deficit. It is a diagnosis of exclusion but the pain the patient experiences may be disproportionately severe to the clinical signs.

4.21 A Acute salpingitis

The false-negative rate for appendicitis is highest in fertile young women and in this group a careful gynaecological history should always be taken, and ultrasound scan and even laparoscopy considered. The history for appendicitis is usually brief, 24–48 hours, and will usually be associated with gastrointestinal symptoms such as anorexia, nausea, vomiting or diarrhoea. A longer history, combined with a vaginal discharge is suggestive of pelvic inflammatory disease, but often this diagnosis is only made at the time of removing a normal appendix.

THEME: UPPER ABDOMINAL PAIN

4.22   G   Pancreatitis

Gallstones are infrequently visible on X-ray but are the commonest cause of acute pancreatitis in the UK. Pancreatitis is also associated with binge drinking or chronic alcohol use, mumps, trauma, and can occur in the postoperative period following upper abdominal surgery. The diagnosis is usually based on the history and very raised serum amylase.

4.23   F   Myocardial infarction

The raised jugular venous pressure indicates right-sided heart failure. Myocardial infarction is an important cause of epigastric pain and an electrocardiogram should always be done.

4.24   H   Perforated peptic ulcer

The assessment of patients with serious and existing disease can be very difficult. This man has recently received methylprednisolone and is at increased risk of upper gastrointestinal bleeding or perforation. The presence of a rigid abdomen and no bowel sounds should always raise the suspicion of bowel perforation. Gas in the peritoneal cavity, shown on an erect chest X-ray or supine lateral abdominal X-ray, is a sign of perforated peptic ulcer disease

4.25   B   Biliary colic

Intermittent epigastric symptoms with a tender right upper quadrant are associated with biliary colic. If accompanied by jaundice, urgent ultrasound scan is required to exclude a gallstone in the common bile duct because of a risk of ascending cholangitis. Acute cholecystitis may occur on a background of biliary colic, but with a presentation including fever, occasionally with rigors, severe right upper quadrant pain and a positive Murphy sign (increased tenderness on inspiration).

4.26   A   Bleeding peptic ulcer

This man is taking non-steroidal anti-inflammatory drugs (NSAIDs) for his arthritis. Gastrointestinal bleeding is a frequent cause of collapse in elderly people. The hypovolaemia is manifested as the postural drop in blood pressure. The patient is not tachycardic because he is taking β-blockers for his hypertension.

THEME: MANAGEMENT OF CONSTIPATION

4.27   A   Isphaghula husk

Normally, patients with diverticulosis are placed on a high-fibre diet. There is some evidence that this lowers the recurrence rate. Unprocessed bran taken with food or fruit juice is the most effective bulk-forming preparation. Patients should be advised to take extra fluid to avoid intestinal obstruction. Finely ground bran in bran bread or biscuits is less effective because it has poorer water retaining properties. Isphaghula is useful in patients who cannot tolerate bran. Several proprietary preparations are available, eg Fybogel, Isogel.

4.28   G   Senna

In this situation it is likely that the codeine and perhaps immobility have caused the constipation. For occasional constipation like this stimulant laxatives such as senna or bisacodyl are indicated. If they are not successful the dose can be increased. Glycerol suppositories are an alternative. These act as rectal stimulant because glycerol is a mild irritant.

4.29   H   Sodium acid phosphate

This man has faecal impaction. Patients are often in great discomfort and require rapid bowel evacuation. Enemas are usually employed, commonly phosphate enemas. They work as osmotic laxatives, drawing fluid from the body and retaining fluid that they are administered with. If they fail manual removal of faeces is required. Larger doses of macrogols (eg Movicol eight sachets daily) can also be used but there will be some delay in the onset of action. They are also osmotic laxatives.

4.30   C   Lidocaine hydrochloride

This man has an anal fissure. The local anaesthetic ointment lidocaine can be applied when necessary before emptying the bowel to try and relieve the pain on defaecation. Local anaesthetic ointments can be absorbed through the rectal mucosa and so long term application should be avoided. They are also potent allergic sensitisers of the anal skin. Many proprietary preparations are available often also containing hydrocortisone and soothing agents. It would be appropriate to give an osmotic laxative such as lactulose although it may take up to 48 hours to act. If the fissure fails to heal glyceryl trinitrate ointment may be tried. Sphincterotomy may be needed.

4.31   B   Continue the PPI and review in 2 weeks

Take a full history and thoroughly examine patients presenting with new-onset dyspepsia (which can be deduced from this scenario as the patient infrequently attends the surgery). A trial of 1 month PPI is usually suggested,[1] though there is inadequate evidence whether this or *H. pylori* testing should be offered first. If there is no response or a relapse, *H. pylori* testing should be carried out. People of any age who present with dyspepsia in association with chronic gastrointestinal bleeding, unintentional weight loss, dysphagia, vomiting, epigastric mass or iron deficiency anaemia (alarm symptoms) should be referred for urgent endoscopy.[1] Also, in those patients over 55 years of age with persistent unexplained dyspepsia (ie 4–6 week history with no obvious cause) without satisfactory response to a PPI and/or *H. pylori* eradication therapy, urgent endoscopy should also be requested.

4.32   B   More prevalent in women

Irritable bowel syndrome is a common condition that affects women more than men. It usually causes symptoms of altered bowel habit but without red flag symptoms such as rectal bleeding. Abdominal pain is often relieved by defecation. Weight loss is not a symptom, and if present should alert the clinician to other underlying pathology.

4.33   B   Prescribe a PPI again

There is a response to treatment here even if relapses occur and therefore the dyspepsia cannot be regarded as persistent. There are no alarm symptoms. Current guidelines[2] recommend offering low dose treatment with a PPI with a limited number of repeat prescriptions. The use of treatment on an as required basis should be discussed to help patients manage their own symptoms. Patients should be reviewed at least annually to discuss medication and symptoms. Retesting for *H. pylori* is not recommended unless there is a strong clinical need.

4.34   B   Endomysium antibody plus IgA level

Coeliac disease affects up to one in 100 people in the UK. Untreated it often results in unnecessary morbidity including growth retardation in children, osteopenia, osteoporosis, anaemia, the development of autoimmune disorders and malignancy (lymphoma and small bowel tumours). The only treatment is a strict life-long gluten-free diet. IgA class anti-endomysial antibodies are very specific, occurring only in coeliac disease and dermatitis herpetiformis The EMA is the initial screening test of choice. It may be negative in the 2% of people with coeliac disease who are IgA deficient. Therefore IgA levels are normally measured at the same time. If the result is positive then jejunal biopsy is offered. If the diagnosis with EMA is uncertain it should be repeated after 6 weeks on a diet that includes four slices of normal bread per day for a maximum of 2 weeks. The test becomes negative within 3–6 months of stopping gluten and is an accepted and reliable marker for compliance with the diet. In coeliac disease the faecal fat level is raised (steatorrhoea) but there are other causes of fat malabsorption, eg pancreatic insufficiency.

4.35   E   None of these

Current guidelines[2] suggest that patients over the age of 45 years with new onset symptoms and patients of any age with alarm symptoms or a strong family history of gastrointestinal cancer should be referred for specialist assessment. This woman has no alarm features such as rectal bleeding, weight loss anaemia or abdominal mass. The diagnosis is irritable bowel syndrome (IBS) and no investigations are needed. Unnecessary referrals and investigations and excess rates of surgery are reported for patients with IBS.

REFERENCES

1. National Institute for Health and Clinical Excellence. Dyspepsia: Management of dyspepsia of adults in primary care (homepage on the Internet), August 2004 (updated 2005 June; cited 2008 April 23). Available from http://www.nice.org.uk/nicemedia/pdf/ CG017NICEguideline.pdf

2. Primary Care Society for Gastroenterology. Irritable Bowel Syndrome: Guidelines for General Practice. November 2001.

Chapter 5
Infectious diseases, Haematology, Immunology and Genetics

QUESTIONS

THEME: INTERPRETATION OF HAEMATOLOGICAL RESULTS

Options

A β-thalassaemia minor

B Acute myeloid leukaemia

C Alcoholic liver disease

D Vitamin B_{12} deficiency

E Chronic lymphocytic leukaemia

F Chronic myeloid leukaemia

G Cytotoxic drugs

H Folate deficiency

I Iron deficiency

J Myelodysplasia

K Old age

L Rheumatoid arthritis

For each set of results below, choose the single most likely diagnosis from the above list of options. Each option may be used once, more than once or not at all.

Normal values

- White cell count (WCC): 4.0–11.0 x 10^9/l

- Neutrophils: 2.0–7.5 x 10^9/l

- Lymphocytes: 1.3–3.5 x 10^9/l

- Monocytes: 0.2–0.8 x 10^9/l

- Haemoglobin (Hb): men 13.5–18.0g/dl; women 11.5–16.0g/dl

- Red cell count: men 4.5–6.5×10^{12}/l; women 3.9–5.6×10^{12}/l

- Mean corpuscular volume (MCV): 76–97fl

- Mean corpuscular haemoglobin (MCH): 27–32pg

- Platelet count: 150–400×10^{9}/l

- Ferritin: 12–200µg/l

☐ **5.1**   **40-year-old woman: Hb 9.0g/dl, MCV 82fl, WCC 8.1×10^{9}/l, platelets 450×10^{9}/l, serum ferritin 300 µg/l.**

☐ **5.2**   **50-year-old man with longstanding epilepsy: Hb 10.1g/dl, MCV 115fl, WCC 3.8×10^{9}/l (lymphocytes 2.5, neutrophils 1.3), platelets 243×10^{9}/l.**

☐ **5.3**   **21-year-old woman, booking visit to antenatal clinic: Hb 9.7g/dl, MCV 71fl, MCH 27pg, red cell count 6.7×10^{12}/l, WCC 6.4×10^{9}/l, platelets 310×10^{9}/l, HbA2 5%.**

☐ **5.4**   **75-year-old woman, investigations for fatigue: Hb 9.4g/dl, MCV 102fl, WCC 4.5×10^{9}/l (lymphocytes 1.8, neutrophils 1.7, monocytes 1.0, myeloblasts 0.1), platelets 190×10^{9}/l.**

☐ **5.5**   **60-year-old man, routine blood test: Hb 10.8g/dl, MCV 87fl, MCH 30pg, WCC 18.4×10^{9}/l, platelets 190×10^{9}/l. Direct antiglobulin test – positive.**

☐ **5.6**   **55-year-old man, routine blood test: Hb 13.8g/dl, MCV 106fl, WCC 6.7×10^{9}/l, platelets 110×10^{9}/l. Blood film – target cells and hypersegmented neutrophils.**

THEME: GENETIC PROBLEMS

Options

A Autosomal dominant inheritance
B Autosomal recessive inheritance
C Chromosomal abnormality
D Polygenic inheritance
E Sex chromosome abnormality
F Sex-linked disorder

For each disorder below, choose the single most likely mode of inheritance from the above list of options. Each option may be used once, more than once or not at all.

☐ **5.7**   **Cystic fibrosis**

☐ **5.8**   **Down syndrome**

☐ **5.9**   **Duchenne muscular dystrophy**

☐ **5.10** **Schizophrenia**

☐ **5.11** **Turner syndrome**

THEME: CHILDHOOD IMMUNISATION

Options

A Adsorbed diphtheria (low dose), tetanus, polio (inactivated) (one injection)

B *Haemophilus influenzae* type b conjugate vaccine (Hib) and meningitis c conjugate vaccine (one injection)

C Diphtheria, tetanus, pertussis (acellular, component), polio (inactivated) and *Haemophilus influenzae* type b conjugate vaccine (adsorbed) (Hib) (one injection)

Meningitis c (meningococcal group conjugate vaccine) (one injection)

D Adsorbed diphtheria, tetanus, pertussis (acellular, component), polio (inactivated) (one injection)

Measles, mumps and rubella (German measles) live (MMR) (one injection)

E Diphtheria, tetanus, pertussis (acellular, component), polio (inactivated) and *Haemophilus influenzae* type b conjugate vaccine (adsorbed) (Hib) (one injection)

Pneumococcal infection (pneumococcal polysaccharide conjugate vaccine, PCV) (one injection)

F Measles, mumps and rubella (German measles) live (MMR) (one injection)

Pneumococcal infection (pneumococcal conjugate vaccine, PCV) (one injection)

G Diphtheria, tetanus, pertussis (acellular, component), polio (inactivated) and *Haemophilus influenzae* type b conjugate vaccine (adsorbed) (Hib) (one injection)
Pneumococcal infection (pneumococcal conjugate vaccine, PCV) (one injection)
Meningitis c (meningococcal group conjugate vaccine) (one injection)

The options above show the vaccine or combination of vaccines that are given at different ages during childhood and adolescence. For each of the ages below select the single appropriate vaccine or combination of vaccines from the list above.

☐ **5.12** 2 months

☐ **5.13** 4 months

☐ **5.14** 13 months

☐ **5.15** Pre-school

☐ **5.16** Adolescence

THEME: ALLERGIC DISORDERS

Options

A   Autoimmune disease

B   Metabolic

C   Pharmacological

D   Type I allergy

E   Type IV allergy

F   None of these

For each of the patients below select the single mechanism from the list above that is likely to be responsible for the development of symptoms. Each option may be used once, more than once or not at all.

☐ **5.17**   A 35-year-old woman says that her migraine headaches are precipitated by drinking red wine.

☐ **5.18**   A 55-year-old woman has troublesome urticaria. She takes aspirin and finds some improvement in the rash when she stops.

☐ **5.19**   A 40-year-old woman has abdominal colic and distension, wind and diarrhoea. Her symptoms improve by excluding milk from the diet.

☐ **5.20**   A 15-year-old boy collapses with anaphylactic shock after eating peanuts.

☐ **5.21**   A 28-year-old man develops a rash on his wrist where he wears his watch.

THEME: HAEMATOLOGICAL CONDITIONS

Options

A Acute lymphoblastic leukaemia
B Acute myeloid leukaemia
C Acute promyelocytic leukaemia
D Chronic lymphocytic leukaemia
E Chronic myeloid leukaemia
F Hodgkin lymphoma
G Monoclonal gammopathy of undetermined significance
H Multiple myeloma
I Non-Hodgkin lymphoma
J Waldenström macroglobulinaemia

For each of the following scenarios, choose the most likely diagnosis from the list of options above. Each option may be used once, more than once or not at all.

☐ **5.22** A 70-year-old retired farmer is found to have a peripheral blood lymphocytosis when a full blood count is done after he presents to his GP with herpes zoster.

☐ **5.23** A 60-year-old African Caribbean man presents to his GP with persistent bony pains. Initial blood investigations reveal an anaemia, raised erythrocyte sedimentation rate (ESR), urea and creatinine, and hypercalcaemia.

☐ **5.24** A pale 4-year-old girl with recurrent infections and ophthalmoplegia undergoes a full blood count. A subsequent bone marrow investigation shows primitive pre-B lymphoblast cells.

☐ **5.25** An HIV-positive man on effective antiretroviral therapy presents with painless lymphadenopathy and fevers, drenching night sweats and weight loss.

☐ **5.26** A pale, thin 50-year-old bank manager presents with tiredness, weight loss and sweating. He has noticed some visual disturbances. Examination reveals splenomegaly. Haematological investigation reveals massive neutrophilia with left shift but low neutrophil alkaline phosphatase score and a high serum vitamin B_{12} level.

THEME: RED BLOOD CELLS

Options

A Fragment cells

B Hypochromia, anisocytosis, poikilocytosis

C Pancytopenia with hypocellular bone marrow

D Pancytopenia with normal bone marrow function

E Raised mean corpuscular volume (MCV) with macrocytosis and normal bone marrow

F Raised MCV with megaloblasts in bone marrow

G Raised red cell count and bone marrow erythroid hyperplasia

H Sickle cells

I Sideroblasts, basophilic stippling

J Spherocytes and reticulocytes

In each of the following clinical scenarios, which one of the above sets of blood/bone-marrow results would represent the most likely findings. Each option may be used once, more than once or not at all.

☐ **5.27** A 56-year-old man with pernicious anaemia.

☐ **5.28** A 63-year-old man with a prosthetic heart valve.

☐ **5.29** A 23-year-old man has previously been admitted for recurrent chest pains and now presents with priapism.

☐ **5.30** A 45-year-old woman with rheumatoid arthritis and a large spleen.

☐ **5.31** A 9-year-old boy with lead poisoning.

☐ **5.32** A 31-year-old Tanzanian man with hookworm infection.

THEME: SEXUALLY TRANSMITTED DISEASES

Options

A Candidiasis

B *Chlamydia trachomatis*

C Gonorrhoea

D Herpes simplex virus

E Human papilloma virus

F Lymphogranuloma venereum

G Primary syphilis

H Secondary syphilis

I Trichomonal vaginosis

For each of the following clinical scenarios, chose the single most likely diagnosis from the list of options above. Each option may be used once, more than once or not at all.

☐ **5.33** A 28-year-old woman has an offensive, profuse, green-grey vaginal discharge. No lesions are visible on speculum examination.

☐ **5.34** There is a painless indurated ulcer on the penis of a 35-year-old man. Smear from the ulcer base is positive to dark-field examination.

☐ **5.35** There is a small painless vulval ulcer in a 29-year-old woman who presents with enlarged lymph nodes in the groin. There are sinuses from the matted nodes.

☐ **5.36** A 24-year-old woman presents with painful urinary retention. She has clusters of small ulcers on the vulva and around the urethra.

☐ **5.37** A 29-year-old man returns from holiday abroad complaining of a milky urethral discharge.

5.38 An 18-month-old boy from a travelling family has unilateral parotid swelling and has signs of meningism.

Select from the list below the single most likely cause.

- ☐ **A** Adenovirus
- ☐ **B** Cytomegalovirus (CMV)
- ☐ **C** Epstein–Barr virus
- ☐ **D** Mumps
- ☐ **E** Rotavirus

5.39 A 70-year-old man has chronic obstructive pulmonary disease.

Select from the list below the single most effective agent for preventing illness from influenza.

- ☐ **A** Amantadine
- ☐ **B** Antibiotics
- ☐ **C** Influenza vaccine
- ☐ **D** Oseltamivir (Tamiflu®)
- ☐ **E** Zanamivir (Relenza®)

5.40 Select from the list below the single situation in which risk assessment either pre-pregnancy or during pregnancy would not be appropriate.

- ☐ **A** Consanguineous couple
- ☐ **B** Family history of atopy
- ☐ **C** Family history of B thalassaemia
- ☐ **D** Family history of polycystic kidneys
- ☐ **E** Older woman

5.41   An 18-year-old woman collapses following a wasp sting. She has a wheeze and stridor and is hypotensive.

Select from the list below the single most appropriate drug or drug combination to treat her.

- [ ] **A**   Adrenaline
- [ ] **B**   Adrenaline and oxygen
- [ ] **C**   Adrenaline, oxygen and chlorpheniramine
- [ ] **D**   Adrenaline, oxygen, chlorpheniramine and hydrocortisone
- [ ] **E**   Adrenaline, oxygen, chlorpheniramine, hydrocortisone and salbutamol

5.42   A 30-year-old male patient's lifestyle may have increased his risk of developing HIV.

Select from the list below the single disease that would not increase your suspicion of HIV.

- [ ] **A**   Extensive molluscum contagiosum
- [ ] **B**   Glandular fever
- [ ] **C**   Hepatitis B
- [ ] **D**   Oral candidiasis
- [ ] **E**   Tuberculosis

ANSWERS

THEME: INTERPRETATION OF HAEMATOLOGICAL RESULTS

5.1   L   Rheumatoid arthritis

Anaemia with a low-normal MCV suggests either partially treated iron deficiency, mixed haematinic deficiency, thalassaemia or anaemia of chronic disease. A high ferritin excludes the first two possibilities. In a 40-year-old woman, chronic disease is the most likely cause and rheumatoid arthritis is a common chronic disease that causes anaemia. A moderately elevated platelet count is also consistent with an inflammatory condition.

5.2   H   Folate deficiency

Macrocytosis, anaemia and neutropenia suggest megaloblastic anaemia, which is caused by deficiency of vitamin B_{12} or folate. Phenytoin impairs folate metabolism and causes actual or functional folate deficiency. Macrocytosis without anaemia is common in patients treated with phenytoin.

5.3   A   β-thalassaemia minor

Minor thalassaemias (β- or α-) cause mild anaemia, with microcytosis out of proportion to the mean cell haemoglobin. They also cause an elevated red cell count, which helps to distinguish them from iron deficiency. Thalassaemia results from decreased production of either α- or β-globin chains of haemaglobin. These are genetic disorders. The homozygous state for α-thalassaemia results in fetal death and for β-thalassaemia produces anaemia requiring regular blood transfusions from an early age. The heterozygous state for β-thalassaemia produces β-thalassaemia minor. The heterozygous state for α-thalassaemia is usually asymptomatic.

5.4   J   Myelodysplasia

Myeloblasts are seen in myeloid leukaemia, leukaemoid reaction, leukoerythroblastic syndromes and myelodysplasia. Myelodysplasia is common in the elderly but is not a feature of normal ageing. Any or all of the cell lines may be reduced. Monocytosis and mild macrocytosis is common and small numbers of myeloblasts may occur. There is no specific treatment, although folate supplements may help. Treatment is symptomatic – transfusion for anaemia, antibiotics for infection, platelet transfusions rarely. The condition may transform into acute myeloid leukaemia.

5.5   E   Chronic lymphocytic leukaemia

Chronic lymphocytic leukaemia is common and is often identified as an incidental finding on blood tests in older people. It may also present with lymphadenopathy, hepatosplenomegaly, bruising, anaemia or recurrent infections. There may be associated thrombocytopenia, anaemia, neutropenia or immunoparesis due to marrow infiltration. Anaemia may also occur due to an associated autoimmune haemolytic anaemia, giving a positive direct antiglobulin (Coombs) test, which may be treated with steroids. Occasionally antiplatelet antibodies also occur.

5.6   C   Alcoholic liver disease

Hypersegmented neutrophils occur in megaloblastic anaemia, uraemia and liver disease. Macrocytosis occurs in megaloblastic anaemia, liver disease, hypothyroidism, myelodysplasia, marrow infiltration, alcohol, pregnancy or haemolysis. Target cells occur in iron deficiency, haemolysis, haemoglobinopathies and liver disease. The common link is liver disease. Alcohol is also directly toxic to platelets.

THEME: GENETIC PROBLEMS

5.7   B   Autosomal recessive inheritance

Autosomal recessive disorders only show in homozygotes. Both parents are heterozygotes with a risk of an affected pregnancy of 1:4. People with the disease usually have normal children unless the partner is heterozygote. Examples include cystic fibrosis, sickle cell disease and thalassaemia.

5.8   C   Chromosomal abnormality

In Down syndrome the commonest disorder is an extra chromosome 21 (trisomy 21). During meiosis a pair of chromosome 21s goes into one cell and none into the other so one gamete has an extra chromosome. A small number are associated with chromosomal rearrangements (translocation) or with mosaicism. In the latter some cells have 46 chromosomes and others 47. This is due to a process of non-disjunction similar to above but, this time, during mitosis after the formation of the zygote.

5.9   F   Sex-linked disorder

These are usually recessively inherited from the mother on the X chromosome. Females are normally carriers so that a male child of a heterozygote mother has a 1:2 chance of inheriting the disease and a female child has a 1:2 chance of carrying the disease. Examples include Duchenne muscular dystrophy, fragile X syndrome, haemophilia and red-green colour blindness. Duchenne muscular dystrophy presents typically by 4 years with progressive difficulty in walking due to muscular degeneration. Sufferers rarely survive beyond the age of 20. Genetic counselling is important.

5.10   D   Polygenic inheritance

Although schizophrenia is known to be a familial disorder there is no simple inheritance pattern but is thought to involve gene combinations. Other examples include atopy, ischaemic heart disease and type 1 diabetes mellitus.

5.11   E   Sex chromosome abnormality

In Turner syndrome the sex chromosomes are usually written as XO, ie deletion of one sex chromosome. Sufferers have female appearance, are of short stature, have absent or rudimentary ovaries and a variety of other abnormalities. Sufferers from Kleinfelter syndrome (XXY) have a male appearance and may only present in adult life with infertility, gynaecomastia and small testis. The extra X chromosome is retained because of a non-disjunction event during meiosis.

THEME: CHILDHOOD IMMUNISATION

5.12 – 5.16   See Table

GP entrants should know the UK vaccination schedule. The full immunisation schedule is given in Table 1.

Table 1: Immunisation schedule in infancy, childhood and adolescence (see British National Formulary)[1]

When	Vaccine	How
2 months (5.12 E)	Diphtheria, tetanus, pertussis (acellular, component), polio (inactivated) and *Haemophilus influenzae* type b conjugate vaccine (adsorbed) (Hib)	one injection
	Pneumococcal infection (pneumococcal conjugate vaccine, PCV)	one injection
3 months	Diphtheria, tetanus, pertussis (acellular, component), polio (inactivated) and *Haemophilus influenzae* type b conjugate vaccine (adsorbed) (Hib)	one injection
	Meningitis c (meningococcal group conjugate vaccine)	one injection
4 months (5.13 G)	Diphtheria, tetanus, pertussis (acellular, component), polio (inactivated) and *Haemophilus influenzae* type b conjugate vaccine (adsorbed) (Hib)	one injection
	Meningitis c (meningococcal group conjugate vaccine)	one injection
	Pneumococcal infection (pneumococcal conjugate vaccine, PCV)	one injection
12 months	*Haemophilus influenza* type b conjugate vaccine (Hib) and meningitis c conjugate vaccine	one injection
13 months (5.14 F)	Measles, mumps and rubella (German measles) live (MMR)	one injection
	Pneumococcal infection (pneumococcal conjugate vaccine, PCV)	one injection
3 years and 4 months to 5 years (5.15 D)	Adsorbed diphtheria , tetanus, pertussis (acellular, component), polio (inactivated)	one injection
	Measles, mumps and rubella (German measles) live (MMR)	one injection
13 to 18 years (5.16 A)	Adsorbed diphtheria (low dose), tetanus, polio (inactivated)	one injection

CHAPTER 5 ANSWERS

THEME: ALLERGIC DISORDERS

5.17   C   Pharmacological

Reports of dietary trigger factors rely on subjective reports from patients. Alcohol, red wine, missing meals and caffeine withdrawal are the most important migraine precipitants.

5.18   C   Pharmacological

Patients usually think urticaria is an allergic condition. In some patients it does develop by a type I allergic mechanism and if the offending agent is obvious then it should be avoided. Most patients are unaware of any obvious allergen and allergy testing is not appropriate. Many people with chronic urticaria are sensitive to salicylates. Salicylates are the active ingredient in aspirin and are found in all plant matter to some extent (fruits, vegetables, herbal supplements, etc). Patients may not be able to tolerate non-steroidal anti-inflammatory drugs. Preservatives used in food and colouring agents (tartrazine) may also worsen urticaria.

5.19   B   Metabolic

Lactose intolerance is the inability to metabolize lactose, a sugar found in milk and other dairy products, because the enzyme lactase is absent or its availability is lowered. There may be a congenital absence of lactase (autosomal recessive). Lactose intolerance also occurs in patients with untreated coeliac disease and sometimes temporarily following gastroenteritis. Some people just do not produce enough lactase after weaning and this is the commonest cause (primary lactase deficiency). This is a complex area and there is also a true allergic hypersensitivity in some people with immediate and delayed responses. There will then often be other symptoms such as urticaria, stridor and shock.

5.20   D   Type I allergy

Type I allergy is a reaction provoked by re-exposure to an antigen. Exposure may be by ingestion, inhalation, injection, or direct contact. The difference between the normal immune response and a type I allergic response is that plasma cells secrete IgE which binds to receptors on the surface of mast cells and blood basophils. Mast cells and basophils coated by IgE are sensitised. The next time there is exposure the same allergen links to the bound IgE on sensitised cells resulting in degranulation and the secretion of pharmacologically active mediators such as leukotriene, and prostaglandin which act on the surrounding tissues. The main effects of these are vasodilation and smooth-muscle contraction. The reaction may be either local or systemic with symptoms varying from mild irritation to sudden death from anaphylactic shock.

5.21   E   Type IV allergy

Type IV allergy is called delayed type as the reaction takes two to three days to develop. The response is not antibody mediated but rather a cell mediated response. The antigen-presenting cells are macrophages which secrete IL-12. This stimulates the proliferation of CD4+ T cells. These produce IL-2 and γ-interferon, further inducing the release of other Type 1 cytokines, thus mediating the immune response. This patient likely has nickel sensitivity and has developed a contact dermatitis.

THEME: HAEMATOLOGICAL CONDITIONS

5.22   D   Chronic lymphocytic leukaemia

This is the commonest adult leukaemia in the UK, accounting for up to 40% of all leukaemias. The median age of diagnosis is 65–70 years and the male:female ratio is 2:1. It generally follows an indolent course and in the early stages patients are asymptomatic but may have splenomegaly. Lymphadenopathy, anaemia, herpes zoster, bacterial infections, autoimmune haemolysis or thrombocytopenia may cause the presentation.

5.23   H   Multiple myeloma

This clinical scenario is suggestive of multiple myeloma, a tumour of bone marrow plasma cells. Bone pain is the commonest presenting feature and is associated with bone destruction and subsequent hypercalcaemia. Plain X-rays may reveal osteoporosis, lytic lesions and evidence of pathological fractures. Renal impairment is common and is usually due to tubular damage caused by Bence Jones proteins. Other causes of renal impairment in myeloma include hypercalcaemia, dehydration, infection, amyloidosis and non-steroidal inflammatory drugs.

5.24   A   Acute lymphoblastic leukaemia

Acute lymphoblastic leukaemias predominantly affect children and may present with clinical features associated with marrow failure, ie anaemia, bleeding and infections. There may also be bone pain, splenomegaly, lymphadenopathy, thymic enlargement and central nervous system (CNS) involvement with cranial nerve palsies as in this case. There is a 60% cure rate with chemotherapy.

5.25   I   Non-Hodgkin lymphoma

Patients with chronic HIV infection are at risk of developing non-Hodgkin lymphoma. As patients with HIV infection live longer, AIDS related malignancies, especially non-Hodgkin lymphoma are becoming more common. It is more aggressive than the non-AIDS related lymphoma.

5.26   E   Chronic myeloid leukaemia

This is a clonal disorder of haemopoietic stem cells characterised by the Philadelphia chromosome which is a balanced translocation between chromosomes 9 and 22. It can occur at any age but the median age is 55–60 years with a median survival of 4–5 years. It is a triphasic disease with most patients presenting during the chronic phase which lasts for 2–7 years. In 50% an abrupt transformation into a blast crisis occurs, when treatment becomes ineffective. The other 50% undergo an accelerated phase which then proceeds to blast crisis more gradually. If there is a massive neutrophilia there may be associated visual disturbances, priapism or deafness.

THEME: RED BLOOD CELLS

5.27   F   Raised MCV with megaloblasts in bone marrow

Vitamin B_{12} deficiency causes a megaloblastic anaemia. Vitamin B_{12} is found in animal products but not in plants – it cannot be synthesised by humans. Therefore, both diet and the ability to absorb vitamin B_{12} are factors to consider if deficiency exists. Pernicious anaemia is caused by atrophy of the gastric mucosa with subsequent reduction in production of intrinsic factor, which is required for the absorption of vitamin B_{12} in the ileum.

5.28   A   Fragment cells

These are damaged red blood cells, which have subsequently resealed their cell membrane. They are incomplete and misshapen. Causes include prosthetic heart valves, renal dialysis and microangiopathic haemolytic anaemias.

5.29   H   Sickle cells

Sickle cell patients experience crises which may be spontaneous or initiated by intercurrent infection, cold or hypoxia. Sickling of red blood cells in small vessels may cause severe pain in almost any site. Chest pain and bone pain are common. Priapism is also seen. Patients may also develop severe neurological sequelae and hyposplenism through recurrent splenic infarcts.

5.30   C   Pancytopenia with hypocellular bone marrow

This patient has Felty syndrome – rheumatoid arthritis (RA) with hypersplenism and pancytopenia. Any cause of chronic splenic enlargement may cause hypersplenism with pancytopenia.

5.31   I   Sideroblasts, basophilic stippling

Lead poisoning leads to inhibition of enzymes involved in haem synthesis, causing anaemia. It also inhibits enzymes that disperse excess RNA and results in abnormal staining of red blood cells on a blood film (discrete blue particles – stippling effect).

5.32   B   Hypochromia, anisocytosis, poikilocytosis

This patient has iron deficiency anaemia. This can result from blood loss, poor dietary intake or decreased absorption. Hookworm infestation of the duodenum is the commonest infective cause worldwide.

THEME: SEXUALLY TRANSMITTED DISEASES

5.33   I   Trichomonal vaginosis

This is a common cause of vaginal discharge, caused by the flagellate protozoan, *Trichomonas*. There is a profuse greenish discharge.

5.34   G   Primary syphilis

Primary syphilis presents as a papule in the mucosa of the lower genital tract, mouth or anorectal region. After 1 week it becomes a chancre – a single painless indurated ulcer. Dark-field examination of a smear from the ulcer base demonstrated *Treponema pallidum*.

5.35 F Lymphogranuloma venereum

Lymphogranuloma venereum is caused by *Chlamydia trachomatis* serotypes L1, L2 and L3. Other serotypes cause a superficial inflammation of the mucosa and are associated with infertility. The classic finding is of matted inguinal lymph nodes with abscess and sinus formation. The primary lesion is a small papule in the lower genital tract which breaks down to form a painless ulcer.

5.36 D Herpes simplex virus

Herpes simplex is a sexually transmitted disease caused by either herpes simplex virus 1 or 2. The lesions are typical small clusters of vesicles but in the moist environment of the vulva they will often appear as small extremely painful ulcers, which can precipitate urinary retention secondary to pain.

5.37 C Gonorrhoea

The commonest sexually transmitted disease causing a milky urethral discharge in men is gonorrhoea. Up to 50% of men and women with gonorrhoea are asymptomatic.

5.38   D   Mumps

This child is unlikely to have been immunised and is presenting with acute mumps. Meningoencephalitis represents the most severe complication of mumps.

5.39   C   Influenza vaccine

NICE has recommended[2] that none of the other drugs is a substitute for vaccination, which remains the most effective way of preventing illness from influenza. Amantadine is not recommended for post-exposure prophylaxis, seasonal prophylaxis or treatment of influenza. Oseltamivir and zanamivir are not recommended for otherwise healthy individuals with influenza. Both are recommended for treatment of at risk patients and oseltamivir for post exposure prophylaxis in at risk patients. This is supposing treatment or prophylaxis can be started within 48 hours of the onset of symptoms or exposure.

5.40   B   Family history of atopy

Atopy is inherited and has a polygenic mode of inheritance. It is very common and there are effective treatments for atopic disorders. The population risk of having a child with a severe or lethal medical condition is around 2%. For a first cousin couple this increases to around 5%. The risks associated with consanguinity are greater if there is a family history of an autosomal recessive condition. If there is a known mutation in the family, the couple can be tested for their carrier status and prenatal diagnosis offered if required. Thalassaemia is autosomal recessive and polycystic kidney disease has both autosomal recessive and autosomal dominant varieties. Pre-pregnancy counselling may be appropriate. Antenatal diagnosis is possible as it is for Down syndrome. The risk of Down syndrome increases in older mothers.

5.41 E Adrenaline, oxygen, chlorpheniramine, hydrocortisone and salbutamol

The management of anaphylactic shock involves securing the airway and laying the patient flat with the legs raised or on the side if there is a risk of vomiting. Adrenaline is administered intramuscularly (see Table 2 for dosages) repeated at 5-minute intervals according to response of blood pressure, pulse and respiratory function. Oxygen should be commenced from the start. An antihistamine (eg chlorpheniramine 10–20mg) is given after the adrenaline by slow intravenous injection and continued for 48 hours to prevent relapse. The action of hydrocortisone 100–300mg by intravenous injection is delayed for several hours so it is only of secondary importance in the acute phase. It should be given to prevent relapse. A nebulised β-agonist such as salbutamol may relieve the wheeze. Assisted respiration or tracheotomy may be necessary.

Table 2: Dose of intramuscular injection of adrenaline for anaphylactic shock[3]

Age	Dose	Volume of adrenaline 1 in 1000 (1mg/ml)
Under 6 months	50μg	0.05ml
6 months–6 years	120μg	0.12ml
6–12 years	250μg	0.25ml
Adult and adolescent	500μg	0.5ml
Self administration (adult)	300μg	0.3ml Some solution remains in the auto-injector after use

CHAPTER 5 ANSWERS

5.42 B Glandular fever

The Royal College of Physicians has published guidelines[4] for HIV testing of patients. HIV testing is strongly recommended for any unusual bacterial, fungal or viral disease. Molluscum contagiosum and candidiasis are unusual in someone of this age; hepatitis B is another blood-borne/sexually transmitted infection like HIV, and tuberculosis is uncommon in the UK. Glandular fever usually occurs between 10 and 25 years and the patient here is only just outside this range. It is caused by the Epstein-Barr virus and diagnosed by the monospot test. However, a glandular fever-like illness, which is negative for the Epstein–Barr virus or a flu-like illness would raise the suspicion of primary HIV infection with a seroconversion illness.

REFERENCES

1. Active immunity. 14.1 *British National Formulary*; 55; 2008

2. National Institute for Health and Clinical Excellence. *Flu prevention – amantidine and oseltamivir.* (homepage on the Internet), September 2003 (cited 2008 April 24). Available from http://www.nice.org.uk/guidance/index.jsp?action=byID&r=true&o=11510

3. Active emergencies. 3.4.3 *British National Formulary*; 55; 2008

4. Royal College of Physicians. *HIV testing for patients attending general medical services.* London: Royal College of Physicians; 2005.

Chapter 6
Musculoskeletal

QUESTIONS

THEME: THE PAINFUL KNEE

Options

A Anterior knee pain in a 15-year-old gymnast with no history of trauma

B Giving way and intermittent swelling

C Intermittent locking and swelling in a patient with osteochondritis dissecans

D Pain along the medial joint line, swelling and inability to extend the joint fully

E Pain over the proximal tibia associated with a tender swelling in a young teenager

Match the conditions listed below to the single most likely clinical picture from the list of options above. Each option may be used once, more than once or not at all.

☐ **6.1** **Anterior cruciate ligament rupture**

☐ **6.2** **Loose body**

☐ **6.3** **Chondromalacia patellae**

☐ **6.4** **Medial meniscus tear**

☐ **6.5** **Osgood–Schlatter disease**

THEME: BACK PAIN

Options

A Bony metastasis

B Central disc prolapse

C Dissecting abdominal aortic aneurysm

D L1–L2 disc prolapse

E L4–L5 disc prolapse

F Mechanical back pain

G Osteoporotic vertebral body crush fracture

H Spinal stenosis

I Spinal tuberculosis

For each of the following clinical scenarios, choose the most likely diagnosis from the list of options above. Each option may be used once, more than once or not all.

CHAPTER 6 QUESTIONS

☐ **6.6** A 33-year-old male company director complains of intermittent lower back pain in the absence of any neurological symptoms or signs. Radiographs are normal.

☐ **6.7** A 43-year-old woman complains of sudden-onset lower back pain radiating down the left leg as far as the heel. She has paraesthesiae over the lateral aspect of the left lower leg and foot. Examination reveals straight leg raising limited to 20° with altered sensation in the above distribution.

☐ **6.8** A 68-year-old woman complains of bilateral buttock and thigh pain associated with back pain after walking 200m; sitting down relieves the pain. She does not have any symptoms at rest. Examination of the back is unremarkable.

☐ **6.9** A 28-year-old woman has severe lower back pain; she is incontinent of urine. Examination reveals loss of sensation over the perineum and straight leg raise is limited bilaterally.

☐ **6.10** A 72-year-old man complains of severe back pain not responding to rest. He is unable to sleep and has lost 6kg over the past 2 months. Examination reveals some tenderness in the lumbar region but no neurological abnormalities.

THEME: PAINFUL HIP IN CHILDREN

Options

A Congenital dysplasia of the hip (CDH)

B Irritable hip syndrome

C Osteomyelitis

D Perthes' disease

E Septic arthritis

F Slipped upper femoral epiphysis (SUFE)

G Still's disease

Match the symptoms and signs listed below with the single most likely condition from the options given above. Each option may be used once, more than once or not at all.

☐ **6.11** A 6-year-old boy complains of intermittent hip pain for several months. Haematological investigations are normal. X-rays show flattening of the femoral head.

☐ **6.12** A 2-year-old girl with a one-day history of increasing hip pain has become unable to weight bear. Her WCC is 22.0 x 10^9/l, with an ESR of 88mm/h and a CRP of 300mg/l. A radiograph of the hip shows a widened joint space.

☐ **6.13** A 12-year-old boy with left groin pain for 6 weeks is noticed to stand with the left leg externally rotated. Examination reveals negligible internal rotation of the hip.

☐ **6.14** A 4-year-old boy complains of right hip pain a few days following an upper respiratory tract infection. Blood tests are as follows: WCC 11.0 x 10^9/l, erythrocyte sedimentation rate (ESR) 10mm/h and C-reactive protein (CRP) 2mg/l.

☐ **6.15** A 5-year-old girl complains of progressively increasing severe pain in her left hip and upper leg for 6 days. She is able to walk but limps visibly. Blood tests are as follows: WCC 19.0 x 10^9/l, ESR 72mm/h and CRP 94mg/l.
X-rays and ultrasound scans of the hip are normal.

THEME: DISORDERS OF THE KNEE JOINT

Options

A   Anterior cruciate ligament injury

B   Gout

C   Meniscal injury

D   Osgood–Schlatter disease

E   Osteoarthritis

F   Osteosarcoma of the proximal tibia

G   Patella bursitis

H   Patella fracture

I   Rheumatoid arthritis

J   Septic arthritis

For each of the following patients, select the single most likely diagnosis from the list of options above. Each option may be used once, more than once or not at all.

☐ **6.16**   A 33-year-old nurse was running for the bus when she tripped and fell over an uneven paving slab. She felt something crack and afterwards was unable to bear weight on the leg. In the Emergency Department, considerable bruising around the knee is noted. She is unable to lift her leg off the couch.

☐ **6.17**   A 50-year-old electrician has a tender fluctuant lump that appears to float under the skin of the kneecap. The overlying skin appears normal.

☐ **6.18** A 55-year-old ex-footballer presents to his GP with a long history of aches and pains in various joints. He has had previous meniscectomies of both knees and since he took part in a charity match last weekend he has had considerable pain and swelling in his right knee. He can barely walk. Examination confirms a large tense effusion within the joint and significant restriction in joint movement. He is otherwise well.

☐ **6.19** A 55-year-old publican presents to his GP with a 24-hour history of acute pain and swelling in his left knee. He has been unable to sleep. Examination confirmed a large effusion in his knee and considerable tenderness. He is known to have history of recent congestive cardiac failure but no significant musculoskeletal symptoms had been documented previously.

THEME: ACUTE HOT KNEE

Options

A Anterior cruciate ligament disruption

B Baker cyst

C Gonococcal arthritis

D Gout

E Lyme arthritis

F Prepatellar bursitis

G Pseudogout

H Rheumatoid arthritis

I Septic arthritis

J Systemic lupus erythematosus (SLE)

For each of the following clinical scenarios, select the single most appropriate diagnosis from the list of options above. Each option may be used once, more than once or not at all.

☐ **6.20** A 29-year-old woman presents with a swollen knee, pyrexia and an erythematous macular rash on her palms and soles of her feet.

☐ **6.21** A 31-year-old woman presents with a hot swollen knee. Her ESR and CRP levels are raised. She has felt generally unwell for a week.

☐ **6.22** A 67-year-old woman presents with a painful, hot, swollen knee. Her joint aspirate is turbid and shows positively birefringent rhomboid crystals on microscopy.

☐ **6.23** A 12-year-old boy presents with a hot swollen left knee, raised ESR, pyrexia and severe pain on passive movement. His joint aspirate is turbid.

THEME: RHEUMATOLOGY

Options

A	Ankylosing spondylitis	F	Psoriatic arthropathy
B	Gouty arthritis	G	Reiter disease
C	Osteoarthritis	H	Rheumatoid arthritis
D	Osteoporosis	I	Scleroderma
E	Polymyalgia rheumatica	J	Systemic lupus erythematosus

For each of the presentations below, select the single most likely diagnosis from the list of options above. Each option may be used once, more than once or not at all.

☐ **6.24** A 53-year-old woman has swan-neck deformities of her fingers and pain in her hips. X-ray examination reveals erosion of the ends of the phalanges.

☐ **6.25** A 23-year-old African Caribbean woman presents with joint pains. She has a red facial rash. On examination, her hands appear normal.

☐ **6.26** A 56-year-old woman presents with knee and hip pain. X-rays of the hips show narrowing of the joint space and osteophyte formation. Examination of the knees demonstrates marked crepitus.

☐ **6.27** A 25-year-old man presents with a long history of low back pain. He is experiencing the acute onset of heel pain. Examination reveals tenderness beneath the calcaneum and a limited range of spinal movements.

☐ **6.28** An elderly woman complains of shoulder stiffness. She cannot brush her hair or apply her make-up due to the stiffness. She denies true weakness. She attends with acute visual loss in the left eye.

CHAPTER 6 QUESTIONS

THEME: PAINFUL UPPER LIMB

Options

A Anterior dislocation of the shoulder

B Colles' fracture

C De Quervain tenosynovitis

D Fractured surgical neck of humerus

E Gamekeeper's thumb

F Posterior dislocation of the shoulder

G Scaphoid fracture

H Supracondylar fracture of the humerus

I Smith fracture

For each of the scenarios below select the single most likely diagnosis from the list of options above. Each option may be used once, more than once or not at all.

☐ **6.29** A 23-year-old man complains of a painful wrist after falling over while drunk. There is tenderness in the thenar eminence and pain abducting his thumb.

☐ **6.30** A 4-year-old girl presents with a painful swollen arm after falling off a pony. The nurse has difficulty taking the radial pulse.

☐ **6.31** A 35-year-old electrician is brought in with a painful upper limb and chest pain following an accident at work in which he received an electric shock.

☐ **6.32** A 67-year-old woman fell while out shopping. She is clutching her arm to her side and complaining of pain.

☐ **6.33** A 31-year-old factory worker complains of a painful arm, which causes difficulty sleeping. There is swelling on the radial side of her forearm above the wrist, with crepitus felt on movement at this site.

6.34 A 40-year-old man has had low back pain for 2 weeks. It radiates to the buttocks and thighs and is worsened by movement. He is otherwise well.

In addition to recommending analgesia, identify from the list below the single most appropriate other initial action.

- ☐ **A** Advise to keep active
- ☐ **B** Bed rest
- ☐ **C** Lumbar support
- ☐ **D** Refer to an orthopaedic surgeon
- ☐ **E** X-ray lumbosacral spine

6.35 A 52-year-old man with rheumatoid arthritis does not respond to sulfasalazine and methotrexate and cannot tolerate gold.

Select from the list below the single most appropriate disease-modifying drug that you can use.

- ☐ **A** Celecoxib
- ☐ **B** Intra-articular corticosteroids
- ☐ **C** Infliximab
- ☐ **D** Naproxen
- ☐ **E** Oral corticosteroids

6.36   A 55-year-old woman has a body mass index of 30. She has bilateral knee osteoarthritis.

Identify from the list below the single therapy that will modify the structural progression of the arthritis.

☐ A   Intra-articular hyaluronan

☐ B   Intra-articular corticosteroids

☐ C   Non-steroidal anti-inflammatory drugs

☐ D   Physiotherapy

☐ E   Weight loss

☐ F   None of these

6.37   A 12-year-old boy has a limp and painful heel that is locally tender when squeezed. He is a keen soccer player.

Which one of the following is the most likely diagnosis?

☐ A   Morton metatarsalgia

☐ B   Navicular osteochondritis

☐ C   Pes planus

☐ D   Plantar fasciitis

☐ E   Sever disease

ANSWERS

THEME: THE PAINFUL KNEE

6.1 **B** **Giving way and intermittent swelling**

The anterior cruciate ligament prevents forward subluxation of the tibia on the femur under normal conditions; its rupture results in instability that is usually associated with a joint effusion.

6.2 **C** **Intermittent locking and swelling in a patient with osteochondritis dissecans**

Loose bodies most commonly arise in knees of patients with osteochondritis dissecans. In this condition there is necrosis of the subchondral bone with subsequent detachment of a fragment of bone and its overlying cartilage. It most commonly affects the lateral surface of the medial femoral condyle.

6.3 **A** **Anterior knee pain in a 15-year-old gymnast with no history of trauma**

Atraumatic anterior knee pain in a teenager is almost invariably due to chondromalacia. More commonly found in girls who exercise regularly.

6.4 **D** **Pain along the medial joint line, swelling and inability to extend the joint fully**

A bucket handle meniscal tear can cause locking (ie inability to fully extend the joint). Medial joint pain suggests a medial meniscus problem.

6.5   E   Pain over the proximal tibia associated with a tender swelling in a young teenager

In this condition, there is traction osteochondritis of the tibial tuberosity at the insertion of the patellar tendon. It tends to occur in active boys and is characterised by anterior knee pain and tender swelling of the tibial tuberosity.

THEME: BACK PAIN

6.6   F   Mechanical back pain

A sedentary lifestyle is the usual cause of mechanical back pain. The absence of any neurological abnormalities is necessary for the diagnosis. Physiotherapy with back-strengthening exercises and postural advice is the mainstay of treatment. Weight loss may be advised if needed and keeping active is important for the recovery process.

6.7   E   L4–L5 disc prolapse

This woman has sciatica. The distribution of her leg symptoms suggests compression of the L5 nerve root which is usually caused by an L4–L5 disc prolapse.

6.8   H   Spinal stenosis

Spinal stenosis causes claudication. The symptoms subside within minutes of sitting down. Assessment of the peripheral circulation is mandatory to exclude any vascular causes. Surgical treatment is by spinal decompression.

6.9   B   Central disc prolapse

This is an emergency. Urgent decompression is required to prevent any irreversible damage. The diagnosis is central disc prolapse.

6.10   A   Bony metastasis

Intractable back pain (ie persisting at rest) in an elderly person is unusual. It suggests a malignant process, particularly if associated with systemic symptoms such as weight loss. Spinal tuberculosis is rare in the UK.

THEME: PAINFUL HIP IN CHILDREN

6.11   D   Perthes' disease

Perthes' disease commonly presents in the 4–9 years age group. It is more common in boys, and often there is a strong family history. The symptoms tend to be relatively minor in the early stages. At a later stage, X-rays may show flattening of the femoral head caused by localised osteonecrosis.

6.12   E   Septic arthritis

This girl has septic arthritis; this condition is characterised by severe pain usually rapid in onset and the child is unable to walk. It occurs most commonly below the age of 4 years. The commonest organism isolated is *Staphylococcus aureus*. High inflammatory markers, along with fluid in the hip joint, suggest the diagnosis confirmed with joint aspiration. The basis of treatment is surgical drainage with adjuvant antibiotic therapy.

6.13   F   Slipped upper femoral epiphysis (SUFE)

Slipped upper femoral epiphysis is found in older children (boys > girls), up to the age of puberty. Classically, the symptoms are insidious in onset, as the displacement is gradual. External rotation of the limb at rest is pathognomonic. A special lateral X-ray view will show the posterior displacement of the upper femoral epiphysis.

6.14   B   Irritable hip syndrome

Irritable hip may follow an upper respiratory tract infection. The pathophysiology is still unknown. The child develops a form of reactive synovitis in the hip with pain and a sterile effusion. Blood tests are usually normal and children are not systemically ill. Aspiration of the hip joint will reveal fluid containing white blood cells but no organisms. Aspiration is also therapeutic as it reduces pain. Recovery usually occurs in 7–10 days without treatment.

6.15   C   Osteomyelitis

Osteomyelitis can be difficult to differentiate clinically from septic arthritis. The pain tends to be more chronic in onset and less severe. In osteomyelitis the child may still be able to walk, which is not the case with septic arthritis.

THEME: DISORDERS OF THE KNEE JOINT

6.16   H   Patella fracture

A patella fracture occurs when the quadriceps contracts against resistance (in this case when the foot was caught against the paving slab). A crack is often heard when the bone breaks. If the extensor mechanism is effectively ruptured (either by rupture of the quadriceps or patellar tendons or by fracture of the patella) the person cannot actively extend the knee or lift the straight leg.

6.17 G Patellar bursitis

Prepatellar bursitis (housemaid's knee) is the inflammation of the pre-patellar bursa, which lies in front of the patella. The normal function of the bursa is to reduce the friction between the patellar tendon and overlying skin when bending the knee. Acute bursitis can be triggered by injury or infection. Chronic bursitis is a longer term problem. Repeated damage to the knee for example from kneeling or work that involves a lot of pressure on the kneecap, as in this case with an electrician, thickens the walls of the bursa, causing irritation.

6.18 E Osteoarthritis

Primary osteoarthritis is often responsible for widespread aches and pains, whilst secondary osteoarthritis is often more specific to joints that have been damaged previously (for example following meniscectomy). Relatively minor trauma (such as playing a game of football) may lead to an acute exacerbation of symptoms and a joint effusion that understandably is uncomfortable and restricts movement.

6.19 B Gout

An acutely swollen and painful knee could be a septic joint but in this case the history of heart disease and his profession should make you wonder about his urate levels. (Some diuretics raise blood urate levels as can alcohol!)

CHAPTER 6 ANSWERS

THEME: ACUTE HOT KNEE

6.20   C   Gonococcal arthritis

This is a form of septic arthritis, although at the time of presentation the joint fluid may be sterile – *Neisseria gonorrhoeae* may still be cultured from the genital tract. Usually the patient has recovered from the initial pyrexial phase and characteristic rash affecting the palms and soles prior to the onset of the large-joint mono/polyarticular arthritis. Treatment involves ciprofloxacin or tetracyclines.

6.21   H   Rheumatoid arthritis

This woman has a monoarticular swelling secondary to underlying systemic disease. Commonly the small joints of the hand are the worst affected but a monoarticular presentation in a large joint may occur. In rheumatoid arthritis both ESR and CRP are raised during active disease. In systemic lupus erythematosus only the ESR is raised.

6.22   G   Pseudogout

This represents an acute synovitis initiated by calcium pyrophosphate crystal deposition in the joint. It often affects elderly women and is very painful. In younger people it may be associated with underlying pathology – Wilson disease, hyperparathyroidism or haemochromatosis. The crystals seen from the joint aspirate in gout (sodium urate) are negatively birefringent under polarised light.

6.23   I   Septic arthritis

Staphylococcus aureus is the commonest cause of septic arthritis. In children *Haemophilus influenzae* must also be considered. Occasionally, other Gram-negative organisms may be involved. The infected joint is hot, swollen and very painful, and usually held in a fixed position as a result of spasm in the surrounding muscles. The patient is usually pyrexial and blood cultures are often positive. Joint aspirate is turbid and should be sent for microscopy and culture. A joint washout and systemic antibiotics are required.

THEME: RHEUMATOLOGY

6.24   H   Rheumatoid arthritis

Rheumatoid arthritis is more common in women than men. Swan-neck deformity and boutonnière deformity of the fingers are characteristic of the condition as is ulnar deviation of the fingers at the metacarpophalangeal joints. The distal interphalangeal joints are usually spared. Radiologically, erosions are the characteristic bone change, along with joint-space narrowing and osteoporosis. Bone destruction is a late finding.

6.25   J   Systemic lupus erythematosus

Systemic lupus erythematosus is nine times more common in women than men. It begins in young adulthood and is more common in those of African and Polynesian descent. The classic rash is a butterfly erythematous facial rash. Joint pain is commonly a prominent feature although examination is usually normal. Serum antinuclear antibodies are positive in almost all cases. Double-stranded DNA antibodies are specific but are seen in only 50% of cases.

CHAPTER 6 ANSWERS

6.26 C Osteoarthritis

Osteoarthritis is a degenerative arthritis affecting the large joints of the lower limbs in particular. The hand and finger joints (especially the distal interphalangeal joints) may be affected, including the carpometacarpal joint of the thumb. Crepitus is a common finding and is usually painless. Radiologically there is narrowing of the joint space and characteristic osteophyte formation.

6.27 A Ankylosing spondylitis

Ankylosing spondylitis is a condition that becomes clinically apparent in late adolescence to early adulthood. It is more common in men than women. Susceptibility is related to HLA-B27 type. Radiologically, an early sign is erosion and sclerosis of the sacroiliac joints, accounting for the back pain.

6.28 E Polymyalgia rheumatica

Polymyalgia rheumatica occurs in patients over 60 years of age, predominantly women. It presents with shoulder girdle pain, stiffness, and only occasionally any weakness. Polymyositis presents with proximal muscle weakness. Polymyalgia rheumatica is associated with temporal arteritis, which may result in sudden visual loss. Treatment in this case is urgent high-dose steroids to relieve symptoms and prevent blindness in the other eye.

THEME: PAINFUL UPPER LIMB

6.29   G   Scaphoid fracture

With a scaphoid fracture there is pain on abducting the thumb. The tenderness is in the anatomical snuffbox area (bordered by the tendons of extensor pollicis longus on the ulnar side and extensor pollicis brevis and abductor pollicis brevis on the radial side) as well as in the thenar eminence. Gamekeeper's thumb is disruption of the ulnar collateral ligament of the thumb at the metacarpophalangeal joint with tenderness at this level.

6.30   H   Supracondylar fracture of the humerus

This is an orthopaedic emergency. In a fracture of the supracondylar region of the humerus, the triceps pulls the forearm posteriorly, resulting in impingement of the brachial artery on the fracture end. The resultant pressure puts the vascular supply to the forearm at risk, hence the poorly palpable radial artery.

6.31   F   Posterior dislocation of the shoulder

Electric shock and epilepsy are two of the commonest associations with posterior dislocation of the shoulder.

6.32   D   Fractured surgical neck of humerus

In older patients a fracture of the shaft of the humerus is possible and can be associated with radial nerve palsy due to injury to the nerve as it passes down the spiral groove. Falls in women of this age may also result in a Colles' fracture of the forearm.

6.33   C   De Quervain tenosynovitis

De Quervain tenosynovitis occurs as a result of repetitive movements such as may be encountered in factory work. Pain is often worse at night. The swelling is of the sheath around the abductor pollicis longus and extensor pollicis brevis tendons at the radial styloid.

6.34   A   Advise to keep active

A review of management guidelines[1] suggests that for simple backache activity should be encouraged as it reduces pain and maintains physical fitness. Absence from work should be discouraged. Prolonged sickness absence makes return to work increasingly difficult. Physiotherapy is beneficial if symptoms persist beyond a few days. Urgent referral is only required if serious spinal pathology is suspected. Lumbar supports should not be prescribed. X-rays should only be carried out if symptoms persist beyond 6 weeks and then only if there is felt to be a specific indication.

6.35   C   Infliximab

Infliximab is a monoclonal antibody directed against tumour necrosis factor-α and is given intravenously. Infliximab can be co-prescribed with methotrexate to prevent loss of efficacy because of antibody formation. Both products halt bone erosion in up to 70% of patients with rheumatoid arthritis, with healing in a few. As a side-effect, some people become autoantibody positive and develop a reversible lupus-like syndrome. Reactivation of old tuberculosis may occur.

6.36   F   None of these

Management objectives[2] for patients with osteoarthritis include education, pain relief, optimising function and modifying structural progression. Intra-articular injections and NSAIDS address pain relief only. Both weight loss and physiotherapy will help with pain and optimise function. There is still insufficient evidence that weight loss will delay structural progression of osteoarthritis of the knee. Although there is no hard evidence to support it, it seems reasonable to advise avoiding obesity and maintaining physical activity as primary prevention.

6.37   E   Sever disease

Sever disease is osteochondritis in the calcaneal epiphysis and typically occurs in children over 8 years. Osteochondritis causes softening and deformity of bone. It can occur in many sites. A rare site in younger children is the navicular bone. Plantar fasciitis causes inferior heel pain in adults. Pes planus is flat feet and common in young children but is generally painless. Morton metatarsalgia is a cause of foot pain in adults caused by entrapment of the interdigital nerve between the metatarsal heads.

REFERENCES

1.   Bandolier. *Back pain*. September 1995 (cited 2008 April 26). Available from http://www.jr2.ox.ac.uk/Bandolier/band19/b19-1.html

2.   Underwood M. *Chronic knee pain in the elderly*. Reports on Rheumatic Diseases Series 5: Hands On. Arthritis Research Campaign February 2005.

Chapter 7
Paediatrics

QUESTIONS

THEME: CHILDREN WITH COUGHS

Options

A Acute epiglottitis

B Angio-oedema

C Asthma

D Bronchiolitis

E Cystic fibrosis

F Diphtheria

G Foreign-body inhalation

H Pertussis

I Retropharyngeal abscess

J Viral croup

For each of the patients below, choose the single most appropriate diagnosis from the list of options above. Each option may be used once, more than once or not at all.

☐ **7.1** A 2-year-old boy with a history of fever and running nose for 2 days is brought to the surgery in the evening with a barking cough and stridor.

☐ **7.2** A 3-year-old boy with a history of raised temperature and coryza for the last 2–3 days develops a paroxysmal spasmodic cough which terminates with a noisy inspiratory sound.

☐ **7.3** A 6-month-old girl is brought to the surgery with dry cough, difficulty in feeding and breathlessness. On examination her chest is hyperinflated, with fine crackles.

☐ **7.4** A 5-year-old girl presents with a sore throat, difficulty in breathing, fever and drooling of saliva. The child is sitting upright, with her mouth wide open.

☐ **7.5** A 6-year-old boy presents with a troublesome nocturnal cough. He gets breathless after sports and his brother suffers from eczema.

☐ **7.6** A 3-year-old boy is brought back to see you because of recurrent chest infections and poor weight gain in spite of voracious appetite. On examination he has nasal polyps.

THEME: ABDOMINAL PAIN

Options

A   Abdominal migraine
B   Acute appendicitis
C   Constipation
D   Diabetic ketoacidosis
E   Hirschsprung's disease
F   Infantile colic
G   Intussusception
H   Irritable bowel syndrome
I   Mesenteric adenitis
J   Pancreatitis
K   Peritonitis
L   Renal calculus
M   Torsion of the testis

For each of the patients below, choose the single most appropriate diagnosis from the list of options above. Each option may be used once, more than once or not at all.

☐ **7.7**   A 3-month-old baby girl is brought in with paroxysmal crying in the evenings. During the paroxysms she draws up her legs.

☐ **7.8**   A 5-year-old boy, with a history of cough and swollen neck glands, presents with abdominal pain. On examination his abdomen is soft, but there is no guarding, and he has tenderness in the right iliac fossa.

☐ **7.9**   A 2-year-old boy is brought with a sudden-onset colicky pain. He looks pale, draws up his legs during a pain episode and passes a red, jelly-like stool.

☐ **7.10** A 4-year-old boy with anorexia, vomiting and a high temperature presents with abdominal pain that initially is central, and then moves to the right iliac fossa.

☐ **7.11** A 7-year-old boy presents with paroxysmal abdominal pain with facial pallor, nausea and vomiting; he is otherwise well. There is a family history of migraine.

☐ **7.12** An 8-year-old boy complains that he has had intermittent colicky abdominal pain and bloated feeling for months. The pain is relieved by defecation; sometimes his stools are normal and sometimes he is constipated.

THEME: MANAGEMENT OF CHILDHOOD ASTHMA

Options

A   Beclometasone 200µg/day
B   Beclometasone 800µg/day
C   Ipratropium bromide 60µg/day
D   Montelukast 5mg/day
E   Prednisolone 5mg daily
F   Prednisolone 30mg daily for 3 days
G   Salmeterol 100µg daily
H   Salbutamol 200µg as required
I   Theophylline 120mg/day

For each patient below, choose the single most suitable option from the above list. Each option may be used once, more than once or not at all.

☐   **7.13**   A 12-year-old boy finds that he increasingly needs to use his β_2-agonist particularly now that he has started rugby and cross-country running.

☐   **7.14**   A 9-year-old girl's asthma has worsened over 1 week in spite of treatment with salbutamol and beclometasone 200 micrograms per day. Salbutamol relieves the symptoms but she is using it frequently. She wakes every night coughing and wheezing.

☐   **7.15**   A 10-year-old boy had his daily dose of beclometasone increased to 400 micrograms one month ago. He still needs to use his β_2-agonist inhaler frequently.

☐   **7.16**   A 4-year-old boy uses beclometasone 400 micrograms per day. In spite of this he regularly needs his β_2-agonist inhaler.

THEME: DEVELOPMENTAL MILESTONES OF CHILDREN

Options

A   6 weeks

B   6 months

C   1 year

D   2 years

E   3 years

F   5 years

From the list of options above select the age at which you would expect a normal child to achieve the developmental stages listed below. Each option may be used once, more than once or not at all.

☐ **7.17**   Sitting unaided

☐ **7.18**   Smiling

☐ **7.19**   Walks up stairs

☐ **7.20**   Dry by day

☐ **7.21**   Cruising around furniture

THEME: FITS AND FAINTS IN CHILDREN

Options

A   Benign paroxysmal vertigo
B   Breath-holding attacks (cyanotic spells)
C   Complex partial seizure
D   Congenital heart block
E   Myoclonic seizure
F   Petit mal
G   Reflex anoxic seizure (pallid spells)
H   Supraventricular tachycardia
I   Syncope

For each patient below, choose the single most likely diagnosis from the list of options above. Each option may be used once, more than once or not at all.

☐ **7.22**   A 10-year-old girl had three episodes of loss of consciousness, the first two at school and the last on a shopping outing at a crowded summer sale. She was well prior to the attacks (all having occurred when she had been standing among a crowd). She had felt dizzy, nauseated and become pale and sweaty before losing consciousness for about 2 minutes. There was no incontinence but twitching of the fingers was noted. On recovery she felt tired.

☐ **7.23**   A 3-year-old had three episodes of vomiting and sudden onset of ataxia over the past 6 months. The attacks were rather short (5–10 minutes) but during them he appeared frightened and pale and had to lie down. After the attack he was back to normal. It was mentioned that he keeps his eyes down or closed when travelling by car or in a lift.

☐ **7.24** A 15-month-old girl has had recurrent episodes of loss of consciousness precipitated by temper tantrums. She is developmentally within normal limits. When upset she starts with a shrill cry, goes blue and floppy, losing consciousness for about 1 minute during which a few jerky movement of limbs may occur.

☐ **7.25** A 7-year-old boy has had four episodes of loss of consciousness over the past 6 months. Two occurred in the morning soon after he woke up when he was noticed to be in a 'dreamlike state' with his head turned to the right and doing 'pill rolling' movements with his hand. This was followed by loss of posture and a generalised seizure lasting 3–4 minutes.

☐ **7.26** A 3-year-old has a history of five attacks of loss of consciousness associated with minor trauma such as knocking of his head or injury to his finger. He becomes pale, loses consciousness and goes floppy, sometimes twitching slightly. During one attack he had a heart rate of 30 beats per minute which rapidly recovered. He regained consciousness rapidly each time.

THEME: JAUNDICE IN CHILDHOOD

Options

A ABO incompatibility

B Biliary atresia

C Breast milk jaundice

D Congenital toxoplasmosis

E Crigler–Najjar syndrome

F Galactosaemia

G Gilbert syndrome

H Glucose 6-phosphodiesterase deficiency

I Hereditary spherocytosis

For each of the following clinical scenarios, select the correct cause from the list of options above. Each option may be used once, more than once or not at all.

☐ **7.27** **A newborn girl develops an unconjugated hyperbilirubinaemia 12 hours after birth associated with a severe metabolic acidosis.**

☐ **7.28** **A baby boy is jaundiced at birth and on examination has a distended abdomen with organomegaly. He also has convulsions.**

☐ **7.29** **A newborn boy develops a progressive conjugated hyperbilirubinaemia with pale stools and dark urine.**

☐ **7.30** **A full-term baby girl develops jaundice on day 3, which continues for 2 weeks. The bilirubin is unconjugated, there is no derangement of other liver function tests and the child remains clinically well.**

CHAPTER 7 QUESTIONS

7.31 A 5-year-old child is brought in by his parents. They are worried that he wets his bed every night. A urine culture is normal and the urine is negative for glucose and protein.

Which one of the following would be the most appropriate management option for this child?

- ☐ **A** Desmopressin nasal spray
- ☐ **B** Oral imipramine
- ☐ **C** Prophylactic antibiotics
- ☐ **D** Reassure the parents that it will settle with time
- ☐ **E** Referral to the specialist for ultrasound and micturating cystourogram

7.32 Which one of the scenarios described below would be most likely to lead to a suspicion of non-accidental injury?

- ☐ **A** Blue discoloration of the back of an infant girl
- ☐ **B** Fractured humerus in a 2-year-old girl
- ☐ **C** Mid-clavicular fracture in a 10-day-old boy
- ☐ **D** Multiple bruises of various age on the shin of a 5-year-old boy
- ☐ **E** Widespread petechial rash in a 2-year-old boy

7.33   A 9-year-old boy has had pericolicky abdominal pain
intermittently over 6 months. It can last for 3–4 hours and
has often occurred in the mornings causing him to miss
school. There are no other worrying features. He is pain free
when seen and examination is normal.

Select from the list below the single most appropriate
course of action.

☐ **A**   Abdominal and renal ultrasound scan
☐ **B**   Barium meal
☐ **C**   Reassure the parents that it will settle with time
☐ **D**   Routine paediatric referral
☐ **E**   Prescribe a proton pump inhibitor

7.34   Which one of the pubertal changes given below does not
normally occur during the age range suggested?

☐ **A**   Age of maximal growth spurt (girls): 12 years
☐ **B**   Menarche (girls): 11–15 years
☐ **C**   Pubic hair development (girls): 10–14 years
☐ **D**   The start of breast development (girls): 12–15 years
☐ **E**   Age of maximal growth spurt (boys): 14 years
☐ **F**   Development of penis (boys): 10–16 years
☐ **G**   Pubic hair growth (boys): 11–16 years
☐ **H**   Testicular enlargement (boys): 9–15 years

CHAPTER 7 QUESTIONS

7.35 Below are abnormalities that can occur in newborn babies. Which single feature in a 2-week-old boy would suggest a high risk of an underlying serious problem?

Assume that each feature is the only abnormality at that presentation.

- [ ] **A** Absent Moro (startle) reflex
- [ ] **B** Failure to regain birth weight
- [ ] **C** Single palmar crease
- [ ] **D** Sticky eye
- [ ] **E** Swollen breasts

ANSWERS

THEME: CHILDREN WITH COUGHS

7.1   J   Viral croup

Viral croup is most often caused by the parainfluenza virus. It commonly occurs in children from 6 months to 6 years of age. Typical features are a barking cough, harsh stridor and hoarseness, usually preceded by fever and coryza. Most cases settle without any intervention, but some children need treatment (oral/nebulised dexamethasone) or occasionally admission for partial airways obstruction. Parents should be warned that the stridor can worsen at night, and they should seek help urgently if they feel the breathing is deteriorating.

7.2   H   Pertussis

Pertussis is a highly infectious form of bronchitis caused by *Bordetella pertussis*. After 2–3 days of coryza, the child develops a characteristic paroxysmal or spasmodic cough followed by an inspiratory whoop (which gives pertussis its common name 'whooping cough'). The cough is worse at night and may be followed by vomiting. Epistaxis and subconjunctival haemorrhage may occur. Symptoms persist for 10–12 weeks. Vaccination or infection do not confer lifelong immunity, but are thought to make subsequent infection less severe.

7.3   D   Bronchiolitis

Bronchiolitis is the commonest serious respiratory infection of infancy. Caused by the respiratory syncytial virus in 80% of cases, it is common in the winter months. Coryzal symptoms precede a dry cough and increasing breathlessness. Wheeze is often present. Feeding difficulty is often associated with dyspnoea. There is no specific treatment and management is supportive.

7.4   A   Acute epiglottitis

Acute epiglottitis is a life-threatening emergency because of the respiratory obstruction. It is caused by *Haemophilus influenzae* type B. The disease occurs in children between the ages of 1 and 6 years. Its onset is often very acute, with a high fever and a toxic-looking child. An intensely painful throat stops the child from speaking and swallowing, and saliva drools down the chin. Soft stridor is present. The child sits immobile and upright with an open mouth to optimise their airway. This is a paediatric emergency.

7.5   C   Asthma

Asthma affects 10–15% of schoolchildren. In childhood it is twice as common in boys as in girls, but by adolescence the ratio is equal. Diagnosis is clinical and depends on a history of recurrent wheeze, cough and breathlessness. In pre-school children the main symptom may be a troublesome cough at night. The diagnosis is supported by a history of a triggering factor or of a personal or family history of atopy.

7.6   E   Cystic fibrosis

Cystic fibrosis is inherited as an autosomal recessive disease. In Caucasians, the carrier rate is 1 in 25. Most children present with malabsorption and failure to thrive from birth, accompanied by recurrent chest infections. Finger clubbing is a feature of established disease. Other features are sinusitis, nasal polyps and rectal prolapse. Older children and adolescents may have diabetes mellitus, cirrhosis or pneumothorax, and boys may be sterile.

THEME: ABDOMINAL PAIN

7.7   F   Infantile colic

Infantile colic is common in the first few months of life. Paroxysmal uncontrollable crying with drawing up of the knees, takes place several times a day, particularly in the evening. The condition resolves by 4 months of age. Advice about how to manage the symptoms is helpful.

7.8   I   Mesenteric adenitis

The associated pain usually resolves within 24–48 hours. It is less severe than appendicitis and tenderness in the right iliac fossa is variable. The disease is most commonly caused by a viral (adenovirus, EBV, Coxsackie B, influenza B) or streptococcal upper respiratory infection. Enteric pathogens such as *Campylobacter*, *Salmonella* or *Yersina* can also be responsible.

7.9   G   Intussusception

Intussusception occurs between 2 months and 2 years of age. It is caused by invagination of the proximal bowel into the distal segment. No underlying intestinal cause is found. A viral illness causing enlargement of Peyer patches may stimulate the lead point. Presenting features are a severe paroxysmal colicky pain and pallor – the child becomes pale, especially around the mouth, and draws the legs up during episodes of pain. A sausage-shaped mass is often palpable in the abdomen. Passage of a stool containing blood-stained mucus, abdominal distension and shock may occur. It should be treated with immediate resuscitation and reduction.

7.10   B   Acute appendicitis

This is the commonest cause of abdominal pain in childhood requiring surgical intervention. Common symptoms are anorexia, vomiting and abdominal pain that is initially central but then localises to the right iliac fossa. Signs are a flushed face with bad breath, fever, tenderness and guarding at McBurney point. Perforation is common in children as the omentum is less developed and fails to surround the appendix.

7.11   A   Abdominal migraine

Abdominal pain usually accompanies cranial migraine, but in children the abdominal pain may be the predominant feature. The pain is usually midline, paroxysmal, with facial pallor. Usually, there is a personal or family history of migraine. Pizotifen can be a helpful prophylactic agent in children with frequent symptoms (to be used under specialist guidance).

7.12   H   Irritable bowel syndrome

This syndrome is associated with altered gastrointestinal motility. There is a positive family history and it is associated with anxiety and stress. Symptoms are bloating, a mucous stool, a feeling of incomplete defaecation, constipation alternating with a loose stool, and the relief of pain by defaecation.

THEME: MANAGEMENT OF CHILDHOOD ASTHMA

These answers are based on recommendations of the British Thoracic Society and Scottish Intercollegiate Guidelines Network.[1]

7.13   A   Beclometasone 200µg/day

For most patients exercise-induced asthma means poorly controlled asthma and in this boy regular preventer therapy should be considered. A low dose of an inhaled corticosteroid is the recommended next step.

7.14   F   Prednisolone 30mg daily for 3 days

In mild to moderate exacerbations of asthma short rescue courses of steroid are helpful to stabilise the condition. The dose is 30-40mg daily for children over the age of 5, 20mg between 2 and 5 and 10mg under 2 years. The medication and compliance should be reviewed and the preventer stepped up if appropriate. Doctors should be aware of the signs that indicate severe asthma. These include being unable to complete a

CHAPTER 7 ANSWERS

sentence in one breath, being too breathless to feed, tachycardia (> 130, 2–5 years, > 120 in children over 5 years) and increased respiratory rate (> 30 breaths/minute in children over 5 years, > 50 breaths per minute, 2–5 years). Wheezing may become less with increasing airway obstruction leading to a silent chest.

7.15   G   Salmeterol 100μg daily

This boy has likely had his betamethasone inhaler increased from a starting dose of 200μg per day. He is now on the maximum recommended dose and the next recommended step in a child over the age of 5 years is to add a long-acting β_2-agonist. High dose inhaled steroids (ie up to 800μg per day) are a later step and a leukotriene receptor antagonist or SR theophylline would be added before this.

7.16   D   Montelukast 5mg/day

In children under 5 years the addition of a leukotriene antagonist is recommended if low dose inhaled corticosteroids do not adequately control the asthma. If this fails specialist referral is required.

THEME: DEVELOPMENTAL MILESTONES OF CHILDREN

7.17   B   6 months

7.18   A   6 weeks

7.19   D   2 years

7.20   E   3 years

7.21   C   1 year

In chronological order most normal children smile at 6 weeks, sit at 6 months, cruise around furniture at 1 year, walk upstairs by 2 years and are dry by day at approximately 3 years. All these stages have ranges but in the question only one normal age has been given for each milestone, eg cruising around furniture is delayed at 3 years and incredibly precocious at 6 months so 1 year is the only possible answer. Major developmental milestones at 6, 12, 18, 24, 36 and 48 months should be learnt. These can be divided into gross motor, fine motor, hearing and language, and social skills.

THEME: FITS AND FAINTS IN CHILDREN

7.22   I   Syncope

Simple syncope results from transient fall in blood pressure due to vasovagal stimulation (dysautonomia syncope) by a variety of stimuli such as pain, fear and standing for a long time, especially in a warm environment. There is a prodrome of dizziness, nausea, buzzing sensation in ears, pallor, sweating and loss of tone followed by loss of consciousness. The electroencephalogram (EEG) does not show epileptic discharges during the episode.

7.23   A   Benign paroxysmal vertigo

This child has typical features of benign paroxysmal vertigo. There is no loss of consciousness, the main feature being transient ataxia. During an attack horizontal nystagmus may be noted. There is increased tendency to have motion sickness.

7.24   B   Breath-holding attacks

This child has typical breath-holding attacks that are precipitated by her being upset and angry. Expiration and apnoea, leading to cyanosis and loss of consciousness, follow the initial cry. The child is bradycardic and may exhibit a few jerky movements. These are self-limiting or respond to behavioural interventions, and cause no lasting damage.

7.25   C   Complex partial seizure

This child has complex partial seizures. There seems to be an aura and some lateralisation at the onset of the seizure that subsequently becomes generalised.

7.26   G   Reflex anoxic seizure

Reflex anoxic syncope first appears around 1 year of age and is precipitated by sudden pain or fright. The child stops breathing and rapidly loses consciousness, becoming hypotonic and pale. There may be a tonic seizure. There is marked bradycardia or a short period of asystole. Recovery is spontaneous and rarely requires intervention.

THEME: JAUNDICE IN CHILDHOOD

7.27   A   ABO incompatibility

Jaundice within the first 24 hours of life is pathological, and often due to haemolysis. As rhesus incompatibility is preventable, ABO incompatibility is now the commonest cause in the UK.

7.28   D   Congenital toxoplasmosis

These signs are suggestive of a congenital infection. Congenital toxoplasmosis results in hepatosplenomegaly, thrombocytopenia and cerebral calcifications. The baby also has convulsions.

CHAPTER 7 ANSWERS

7.29   B   Biliary atresia

Biliary atresia is a congenital defect in which there are variable degrees of abnormality of the biliary tract resulting in a progressive obstructive jaundice. Surgical intervention is invariably necessary.

7.30   C   Breast milk jaundice

This scenario is highly suggestive of breast milk jaundice especially since liver function tests and the clinical condition are normal. It is caused by hormonal interaction (5-β-pregnane-3-α-20 β-diol) of breast milk with hepatic enzymes, and will go away if left untreated. The bilirubin is mainly unconjugated, and no kernicterus has been reported with this kind of jaundice.

7.31   D   Reassure the parents that it will settle with time

About 15% of children have enuresis at the age of 5 years: 5% of 10-year-olds and 1% of 15-year-olds still wet the bed. The boy:girl ratio is 2:1. Treatment is not undertaken until a child is 6 years of age. In this case, both the child and parents should be given an explanation and reassurance. Star charts and an enuresis alarm are effective in motivated children. Desmopressin tablets, can be prescribed for children over 7 years of age for short-term intervention (eg school trips or combined with other measures as part of training) but *BNFC* guidance should be followed.[2] Intranasal demopressin is no longer recommended because it has a greater risk of hyponatraemia, water intoxication and convulsions. Imipramine is avoided due to its side-effects and the risk of overdose.

7.32   B   Fractured humerus in a 2-year-old girl

A mid-clavicular fracture in a 10-day-old baby is most likely to be the result of a difficult delivery and a history of the mode of birth should be taken. Although a facial petechial rash may be a sign of smothering, it could be due to a cough, as in whooping cough. A generalised petechial rash should raise the suspicion of idiopathic thrombocytopenic purpura or meningococcal septicaemia. A blue discoloration on the back of an infant is Mongolian blue spot. It is a harmless congenital blue marking on the buttock or sacrum and is commonly mistaken for abuse. Bruises, of different ages, in a 5-year-old child are a normal finding, but would be suspicious if the child was less than 7 months of age. The diagnosis of child abuse is difficult and requires a holistic approach. However, certain injuries are said to be pathognomonic of abuse. The reported incidence of abuse with humeral fractures seems high. Spiral or oblique fractures in particular, in children under the age of 3, more often occur as a result of abuse. Although not pathognomonic of child abuse, a humeral fracture in a young child should lead to further investigation of its cause.[3]

7.33   C   Reassure the parents that it will settle with time

In the majority (approximately 90%) recurrent abdominal pain in childhood is due to functional illness. In this situation the presence of possible school refusal makes a functional diagnosis more likely. The further away the pain is from the umbilicus the more likely it is to have an organic cause. The parents should be reassured, an MSU sent, the weight recorded and follow up offered. Should any worrying features develop then further investigations/referral may follow.

7.34   D   The start of breast development (girls): 12–15 years

Breast development typically starts at 8–12 years of age. This is usually the first sign of pubertal development in a girl and starts before menarche and pubic hair development.

7.35   A   Absent Moro (startle) reflex

The Moro reflex, also known as the startle reflex, is one of the infantile reflexes. It is normally present in all infants up to 4 or 5 months of age, and its absence indicates a serious disorder of the motor system. An absent or inadequate Moro response on one side is found in infants with hemiplegia, brachial plexus palsy, or a fractured clavicle. Failure to regain birth weight is usually due to a feeding problem or minor intercurrent illness. Nevertheless weight should be monitored. Sticky eye is usually due to a blocked tear duct. It should be swabbed to exclude ophthalmia neonatorum and bathed with boiled water. Antibiotics should be avoided unless clearly infected. Single palmar crease is common and should raise no alarm unless other features of a genetic abnormality are present (eg Down syndrome). Swollen breasts are due to maternal hormones.

REFERENCES

1.   British Thoracic Society and Scottish Intercollegiate Guidelines Network. *British Guideline on the Management of Asthma* (homepage on the Internet), February 2003 (updated July 2007; cited 2008 April 28). Available from http://www.sign.ac.uk/guidelines/fulltext/63/index.html

2.   *Drugs for urinary frequency, enuresis and incontinence.* 7.2.2. British National Formulary for children; 2007.

3.   Williams R, Hardcastle N. Humeral fractures and non-accidental injury in children. Emerg Med J. 2005 February; 22(2): 124.

Chapter 8
Pharmacology and Therapeutics

QUESTIONS

THEME: DRUGS IN PREGNANCY

Options

A Alcohol

B Diclofenac

C Isotretinoin

D Ramipril

E Simvastatin

F Tetracycline

G Trimethoprim

H Warfarin

For each of the adverse effects described below, choose the single most likely medication taken during pregnancy from the list of options above. Each option may be used once, more than once or not at all.

☐ **8.1** Children may have discoloured teeth.

☐ **8.2** It may cause small head size and a hypoplastic nose. In late pregnancy placental and fetal haemorrhage is a risk.

☐ **8.3** It causes severe facial, cardiovascular and CNS abnormalities. Effective contraception should be taken for 1 month before, during and for 1 month after treatment.

☐ **8.4** It causes intrauterine growth retardation, facial abnormalities and cognitive impairment.

THEME: DRUGS AND RENAL IMPAIRMENT

Options

A Amoxycillin

B Aspirin

C Cefalexin

D Furosemide

E Metformin

F Metoclopramide

G Naproxen

H Nitrofurantoin

I Ramipril

J Simvastatin

For each statement below select the single drug from the list above to which it applies. Each option may be used once, more than once or not at all.

☐ **8.5** Increases the risk of lactic acidosis

☐ **8.6** Ineffective because of inadequate urinary concentrations

☐ **8.7** High doses often required

☐ **8.8** Increased risk of extrapyramidal reaction

☐ **8.9** Monitor for hyperkalaemia

THEME: SIDE-EFFECTS OF DRUGS

Options

A Amiodarone

B Aspirin

C Atenolol

D Carbimazole

E Chlorpromazine

F Erythromycin

G Levodopa

H Lisinopril

I Lithium

J Metformin

K Sulfasalazine

L Verapamil

For each group of side-effects below, choose the most likely causative agent from the list of options above. Each option may be used once, more than once or not at all.

☐ **8.10** Cold hands and feet, fatigue, impotence

☐ **8.11** Peripheral neuropathy, pulmonary fibrosis, hyperthyroidism

☐ **8.12** Postural hypotension, involuntary movements, nausea, discoloration of the urine

☐ **8.13** Thirst, polyuria, tremor, rashes, hypothyroidism

☐ **8.14** Sore throat, rash, pruritus, nausea

☐ **8.15** Parkinsonian symptoms, abnormal face and body movements, restlessness and rhythmic, involuntary movements of the tongue, face and jaw.

THEME: WARNINGS FOR SPECIFIC DRUGS

Options

A   Avoid exposure of the skin to direct sunlight

B   May cause blue-tinted vision

C   May reduce effect of contraceptive

D   Must avoid alcoholic drinks

E   Must be taken on an empty stomach

F   Must be taken with food

G   Not to be stopped without doctor's advice

H   Not to be taken with antacids

I   Not to be taken with iron tablets

J   Take with a full glass of water at least 30 minutes before breakfast and remain upright until after breakfast

For each of the drugs below, choose the single best advice from the list of options above. Each option may be used once, more than once or not at all.

☐ **8.16**   Metronidazole

☐ **8.17**   Ferrous sulphate

☐ **8.18**   Prednisolone

☐ **8.19**   Alendronate

☐ **8.20**   Amoxicillin

THEME: DRUGS IN CHILDHOOD

Options

A Aminophylline

B Aspirin

C Azithromycin

D Benzylpenicillin

E Cefotaxime

F Erythromycin

G Griseofulvin

H Ibuprofen

I Isoniazid

J Terbinafine

K Tetracyclines

For each of the clinical scenarios below, select the correct drug from the list of options above. Each option may be used once, more than once or not at all.

☐ **8.21** It is recommended as first-line empirical intravenous treatment in bacterial meningitis where the cause of infection is not known.

☐ **8.22** It is not recommended for analgesic or antipyretic use in children under 12 years of age.

☐ **8.23** This is the only licensed systemic agent for dermatophyte skin infection in children under 12 years.

☐ **8.24** It can be used to treat acne vulgaris in children under the age of 12 years.

THEME: DRUG INTERACTIONS

Options

A Amoxicillin

B Bezafibrate

C Bumetanide

D Cimetidine

E Ciprofloxacin

F Colestyramine

G Ezetimibe

H Minocycline

I Protamine sulphate

J Spironolactone

K Vitamin K

From the list above select the drug most likely to be responsible for the adverse event described in the following case scenarios. Each option may be used once, more than once or not at all.

☐ **8.25** A 57-year-old woman with chronic asthma, who is taking theophylline, is being treated for dysuria and frequency by her GP. She is brought into the Emergency Department with a pulseless ventricular tachycardia.

☐ **8.26** A 61-year-old man with a prosthetic heart valve is taking warfarin. In hospital for an angiogram, his international normalised ratio (INR) is noted to be 6.9 and he has a severe nosebleed. The house officer starts treatment without consulting his senior colleagues. Twelve hours later the patient has a new cardiac murmur and severe heart failure.

☐ **8.27** A 43-year-old man is taking ciclosporin following renal transplantation. He is treated for a 'chest infection'. Three days later, after admission to hospital, he is noted to have severe renal failure.

☐ **8.28** A 67-year-old man, who is taking digoxin for atrial fibrillation, is brought into the Emergency Department with severe muscular weakness. There are multiple ventricular ectopic beats and small T waves on the electrocardiogram (ECG).

☐ **8.29** A 64-year-old man with non-insulin-dependent diabetes usually well controlled with metformin and diet is brought into the Emergency Department unconscious. On testing, his bedside glucose reading (BM stix) is 2.0. He has recently started a new medicine prescribed by his GP.

☐ **8.30** A 55-year-old man has ischaemic heart disease. His serum cholesterol level has not been adequately controlled with simvastatin. He now has muscle pain and weakness and a markedly raised creatine kinase level.

8.31   **A 25-year-old woman is breast feeding.**

Select from the list below the single drug that she should not take.

- [ ] **A**   Beclometasone inhaled
- [ ] **B**   Combined oral contraceptive
- [ ] **C**   Erythromycin
- [ ] **D**   Levothyroxine
- [ ] **E**   Warfarin

8.32   **Approximately 15% of general practice consultations are for skin problems.**

Select from the list below the single drug that should be discontinued immediately should a skin rash appear.

- [ ] **A**   Allopurinol
- [ ] **B**   Amiodarone
- [ ] **C**   Atorvastatin
- [ ] **D**   Risperidone
- [ ] **E**   Sodium valproate

8.33   **A 27-year-old professional man, presently stable on 20mg fluoxetine for mild depression, is seeking advice about resuming driving his car.**

Which one recommendation by the DVLA applies in this case?

- [ ] **A**   A licence is usually refused
- [ ] **B**   He can resume driving if there is no other complication
- [ ] **C**   He should refrain from driving for 6 months
- [ ] **D**   He should refrain from driving for 12 months
- [ ] **E**   He should refrain from driving pending a medical report

8.34 Thyroid function tests are routinely monitored in patients taking certain drugs. A result shows an evelated serum free-T4 but a normal level of thyrotropin stimulating hormone (TSH).

Select from the list below the single most likely drug to be responsible for this result.

- [ ] **A** Amiodarone
- [ ] **B** Carbimazole
- [ ] **C** Levothyroxine
- [ ] **D** Lithium
- [ ] **E** Propylthiouracil

8.35 A 55-year-old man has severe chronic liver disease.

Select from the list below the single drug that can be safely given.

- [ ] **A** Bendroflumethiazide
- [ ] **B** Diamorphine
- [ ] **C** Naproxen
- [ ] **D** Nitrazepam
- [ ] **E** Penicillin V

ANSWERS

THEME: DRUGS IN PREGNANCY[1]

8.1 F Tetracycline

Tetracycline is deposited in teeth and in growing bone as it binds to calcium, and can cause dental staining and growth defects, and altered bone growth. Tetracyclines are contraindicated in pregnant or breastfeeding women and in children < 12 years.

8.2 H Warfarin[2]

If possible, warfarin should be avoided during pregnancy. If warfarin is essential, it should be avoided at least during the first trimester (because of teratogenicity) and from about 4 weeks before delivery to reduce risk of haemorrhagic complications. Unfractionated heparin or low molecular weight heparin could be substituted when appropriate because these agents do not cross the placenta.

8.3 C Isotretinoin

Isotretinoin is a synthetic retinoid that is very effective in severe acne, hence most women taking it will be of child-bearing age. Patients should take a pregnancy test before starting isotretinoin and take a monthly pregnancy test while on the medication. Effective contraception (oral progestogen-only contraception is not considered effective) should be used. Two forms of birth control are often recommended even if one of the forms of contraception, is hormonal, starting 1 month before treatment, during the entire course of treatment, and for 1 month after ceasing treatment.

8.4   A   Alcohol

Alcohol causes the fetal alcohol syndrome (FAS). This is not a uniform clinical picture, but a spectrum of disorders, varying in severity. There are 3 main components of FAS:

*   Facial abnormalities, especially in the mid-facial area

*   Intrauterine growth retardation and failure to catch up

*   Mental problems of cognitive impairment, learning disabilities and impulsiveness

THEME: DRUGS AND RENAL IMPAIRMENT[3]

8.5   E   Metformin

It is not clear how metformin causes lactic acidosis but it interferes with the production and clearance of lactate. Renal insufficiency results in lowered clearance of both lactate and metformin, increasing the risk of lactic acidosis. Additionally, any condition leading to tissue hypoxia may contribute to the development of lactic acidosis, because pyruvate is converted to lactate (the alternative pathway in the Krebs cycle) during tissue hypoxia. Thus, in addition to renal failure, the following co-morbid conditions can contribute to lactate accumulation: pulmonary disease, liver failure, cardiac impairment, shock states, severe dehydration, and microvascular disease.

8.6   H   Nitrofurantoin

Insufficient drug is filtered to be effective in a urinary infection. Prolonged use is associated with neuropathies due to drug accumulation. Ciprofloxacin, a cephalosporin or trimethoprim can be used.

8.7   D   Furosemide

High doses (up to 2g daily) are often needed to achieve significant diuresis because the drug acts directly on the loop of Henle. In renal disease there has been significant renal destruction. High dose intravenous furosemide in renal failure can cause ototoxicity.

8.8   F   Metoclopramide

Metoclopramide is an antiemetic whose activities closely resemble the phenothiazines and hence can induce acute dystonic reactions involving facial and skeletal muscle spasms and oculogyric crises. The risk is increased in renal failure.

8.9   I   Ramipril

ACE inhibitors cause potassium retention, as does renal failure.

THEME: SIDE-EFFECTS OF DRUGS

8.10   C   Atenolol

Use of β-blockers is often limited by their side-effects. Fatigue and impotence, in particular, are commonly described. In fact, impotence is a potential side-effect of most antihypertensives, including angiotensin-converting enzyme (ACE) inhibitors, thiazide diuretics and some calcium channel blockers (eg nifedipine and amlodipine). It is quite likely that, in many cases, the main cause for erectile dysfunction is the hypertension and not the drug.

8.11   A   Amiodarone

Amiodarone can cause many adverse effects, which limits the use of this otherwise versatile antiarrhythmic. It may affect many organs:

- Lungs: alveolitis, fibrosis, pneumonitis
- Thyroid: hyperthyroidism, hypothyroidism (both common)
- Liver: jaundice, hepatitis, cirrhosis, raised transaminases
- Nervous system: nightmares, neuropathy, headache, ataxia, tremor
- Musculoskeletal: myopathy, arthralgia
- Eyes: reversible corneal microdeposits, optic neuritis (rare)
- Skin: photosensitivity, dermatitis, persistent slate-grey discoloration (rare)
- Heart: bradycardia, conduction disturbances

8.12   G   Levodopa

Levodopa-containing drugs often cause gastrointestinal disturbance, particularly nausea, which may be minimised by taking the tablets on a full stomach. Urine and other body fluids may be stained red. Cardiovascular effects include postural hypotension, which may limit the dose that the patient will tolerate (severe postural hypotension should raise the possibility of multisystem atrophy as a cause of parkinsonism and autonomic failure). Neurological side-effects may occur early (dizziness, agitation and insomnia) or late (dyskinesias, psychosis and hallucinosis). Dyskinesias may occur with peak levodopa levels or with 'wearing-off'.

8.13   I   Lithium

Thirst, polyuria, fine tremor and weight gain are common side-effects of lithium. Lithium may induce nephrogenic diabetes insipidus after prolonged usage. Patients may develop goitre with lithium and some will go on to become hypothyroid. Lithium is reabsorbed in the kidney by the same mechanism as sodium and water. Patients may develop lithium toxicity if they become dehydrated or hyponatraemic. Early lithium toxicity causes coarse tremor, agitation and twitching. Later features are coma, convulsions, arrhythmias and renal failure. Treatment is supportive with hydration and anti-convulsants as required. Dialysis is occasionally needed in severe cases.

8.14   D   Carbimazole

Nausea and gastrointestinal upset are common, non-specific side-effects of carbimazole. Rashes and pruritus are also quite common and are allergic in origin. A patient who develops a rash should be switched to propylthiouracil. Agranulocytosis and neutropenia is a rare idiosyncratic reaction to carbimazole. Patients should be specifically counselled to report any sign of infection immediately, especially a sore throat, and an urgent full blood count should be done. Agranulocytosis is reversible on stopping the drug.

8.15   E   Chlorpromazine[4]

The extrapyramidal symptoms depend on dose, the type of drug and individual susceptibility. Parkinsonian symptoms are more common in adults and may appear gradually. These settle if the drug is withdrawn and may be suppressed by anti-muscarinic drugs. Dystonia (abnormal face and body movements) and dyskinesia occur more frequently in younger patients sometimes after only a few doses. Akasthisia (restlessness) is more common when large initial doses are used and may resemble an exacerbation of the condition being treated. Tardive dyskinesia (rhythmic, involuntary movements of the tongue, face and jaw) usually develops on long-term treatment or with high doses. It may be irreversible. Fine movements of the tongue are an early sign and consideration should be given to withdrawing the drug at that stage.

THEME: WARNINGS FOR SPECIFIC DRUGS

8.16   D   Must avoid alcoholic drinks

Metronidazole inhibits aldehyde dehydrogenase and causes acetaldehyde to accumulate in the blood. A disulphiram-like reaction occurs and patients may complain of facial flushing, throbbing headache and palpitations. A patient taking metronidazole orally should abstain from drinking alcohol while taking the drug and for 48 hours after stopping.

8.17   H   Not to be taken with antacids

Iron is best absorbed in the presence of vitamin C, but inhibited by milky drinks or tannins in tea. Antacids inhibit the absorption of most medications, due to chelation by calcium. This is particularly the case with tetracycline antibiotics, which bind to calcium in the body (this is how they stain teeth) or ingested milk. Patients should be advised to avoid taking antacids or other calcium supplements at the same time of day as other medication.

8.18   G   Not to be stopped without doctor's advice

Prolonged use of prednisolone depresses the ability of the body's adrenal glands to produce corticosteroids. Abruptly stopping can cause symptoms of corticosteroid insufficiency, with nausea, vomiting and possible shock. Therefore, withdrawal of prednisolone is usually gradual, which also reduces the risk of an abrupt flare of the disease under treatment

8.19   J   Take with a full glass of water at least 30 minutes before breakfast and remain upright until after breakfast

Alendronate is associated with a risk of oesophageal spasm, pain, ulcers and strictures. Patients may reduce this risk by following the advice given in the question. This certainly limits compliance with an otherwise useful drug. Patients should also be warned to stop the drug and seek medical attention if they develop oesophageal symptoms.

8.20   C   May reduce effect of contraceptive

Amoxicillin and other broad-spectrum antibiotics may cause reduced oral contraceptive efficacy. This is due to the loss of bowel flora that normally recycle ethinyloestradiol from the large bowel. The risk is relatively small but patients should use barrier methods during the course of antibiotics and for a week afterwards. Rifampicin, on the other hand, is a potent hepatic enzyme inducer and almost certainly renders standard dose contraceptives useless.

THEME: DRUGS IN CHILDHOOD

8.21   E   Cefotaxime

Cefotaxime is now recommended by both UK and US academic panels as the drug of choice for empirical treatment in bacterial meningitis. Ceftriaxone is an alternative. In younger age groups, amoxicillin should be added to cover against *Listeria* infection. If parenteral treatment is needed in the community, some local protocols still recommend benzyl penicillin.

8.22   B   Aspirin

This is due to the risk of Reye's syndrome. Reye's syndrome is fatty necrosis of the liver that can lead to fulminant liver failure and encephalopathy and is thought to be caused by certain drugs, especially aspirin.

8.23   F   Griseofulvin

There is a particular need for systemic antifungal treatment in tinea capitis. Although terbinafine is a more effective drug it is not licensed for use in children, but many doctors do use it. Griseofulvin is licensed but finding a suitable preparation for children can be problematic as it is only easily available in tablet form. Tinea capitis is a dermatophyte infection. Dermatophyte infections elsewhere in children can be treated with topical preparations.

8.24   F   Erythromycin

Tetracyclines are normally the first choice systemic therapy for acne but they have long been associated with the staining and malformation of teeth and are not recommended for younger children. Erythromycin or trimethoprim are suitable alternatives and treatment is normally given for several months.

THEME: DRUG INTERACTIONS

8.25   E   Ciprofloxacin

Ciprofloxacin increases the plasma levels of theophylline, leading to an increased risk of cardiac arrhythmias. If the two drugs are to be used together, the theophylline dose should be reduced and the plasma theophylline levels closely monitored.

8.26   K   Vitamin K

The house officer has presumably given vitamin K. A symptomatic patient with a high INR and a prosthetic heart valve should have a controlled reduction of the INR. If the INR drops below the required therapeutic level the patient is at risk of clots forming on the prosthetic valve, leading to valve failure and embolic phenomena. Reduction of the INR in these patients should be discussed with the haematology department.

8.27   E   Ciprofloxacin

Ciclosporin is a calcineurin inhibitor. It is may be used to suppress the immune system and has a major role in post-transplant immunosuppression to prevent and treat graft-versus-host disease. It is also markedly nephrotoxic and requires drug level monitoring to ensure a therapeutic range is achieved. Drugs such as quinolones (ciprofloxacin), vancomycin, co-trimoxazole and aminoglycosides increase the risk of ciclosporin toxicity. Macrolides directly increase plasma ciclosporin levels.

8.28   C   Bumetanide

Digoxin toxicity may produce cardiac arrhythmias or heart block. Hypokalaemia caused by a potent loop diuretic may predispose a patient to digoxin toxicity. Correction of the electrolyte disturbance and withdrawal of digoxin will usually correct the situation. For those with life-threatening digoxin overdose, specific digoxin antibodies may be given.

8.29   D   Cimetidine

Cimetidine inhibits the renal elimination of metformin, leading to higher plasma levels. This in turn may lead to hypoglycaemia.

8.30   B   Bezafibrate

Combination of a fibrate with a statin carries an increased risk of side-effects. Muscle pain, myositis and rarely rhabdomyolisis causing renal failure and myoglobinuria may occur. Patients should be warned and monitoring of creatine kinase considered.

8.31   B   Combined oral contraceptive[5]

The combined oral contraceptive should be avoided because it interferes with lactation. Progestogen-only contraceptives do not adversely affect lactation. With inhaled beclometasone and levothyroxine the amounts in breast milk are too small to be harmful. Erythromycin can be safely given to infants. If infants are vitamin K deficient then there is an increased risk of haemorrhage if the mother takes oral anticoagulants. Warfarin is regarded as safe but phenindione should be avoided and the manufacturer of acenocoumarol (nicoumalone) recommends prophylactic vitamin K for the baby.

8.32   A   Allopurinol

Most drugs have skin rash listed as one of their side-effects. Diagnostic certainty can be difficult with many rashes that present acutely in general practice. It is difficult to decide what to do if somebody develops a new rash while taking one, or more usually, several drugs. For instance many patients are incorrectly labelled penicillin allergic because they happen to develop a rash while taking penicillin. It may be very important for the patient that they continue all the drugs presented here. All are reported to cause rashes, some serious such as Stevens–Johnson syndrome and toxic epidermal necrolysis with atorvastatin and sodium valproate, fortunately rare. Rash is the commonest side effect with allopurinol but because of the risk of allopurinol hypersensitivity syndrome (ASH) , which is commonly fatal, therapy should be withdrawn immediately. ASH consists of a rash, including toxic epidermal necrolysis, erythema multiforme or a diffuse macropapular or exfoliative dermatitis and worsening renal function. There may also be fever, leucocytosis and eosinophilia. If the rash is mild the drug can be re-introduced cautiously but should be stopped immediately if there is a recurrence.[6]

8.33   B   He can resume driving if there is no other complication

A person with uncomplicated depression or anxiety who is stable on treatment can return to driving, providing there is no complication from the medication prescribed, eg medications with a sedative side-effect. Fluoxetine is not a sedative antidepressant. In severe depression or severe anxiety the DVLA should be informed and driving stopped, pending medical recommendation (a period of stability is required before driving can be resumed). In mild dementia the recommendations are similar but subject to annual review. In cases of acute psychosis or alcohol or opioid dependency, a person's licence is revoked for 12 months. Drug abusers can only resume driving after a drug-free period of 12 months. Regulations for driving a heavy or public vehicle are more stringent, and the counterpart of 12 months in this category is usually 3 years.[7]

8.34   A   Amiodarone

Amiodarone causes both hypothyroidism and hyperthyroidism. It also inhibits peripheral conversion of levothyroxine (T4) to triiodothyronine (T3), and may cause isolated biochemical changes (increase in serum free-T4, free-T3 being slightly decreased or even normal) in clinically euthyroid patients. There is no reason in such cases to discontinue amiodarone treatment if there is no clinical or further biological (ie TSH) evidence of thyroid disease. Lithium causes hypothyroidism. Levothyroxine is used in replacement therapy for hypothyroidism, and carbimazole or propylthiouracil are used to treat hyperthyroidism. In all of these changes to free-T4 should be accompanied by changes to TSH.

8.35   E   Penicillin V

Penicillin is one of the safest antibiotics for patients with liver disease. In severe liver disease many drugs can further impair cerebral function and precipitate encephalopathy. These include sedatives (nitrazepam), opioid analgesics (diamorphine) and drugs producing hypokalaemia (bendroflumethiazide). NSAIDs (naproxen) increase the risk of gastric bleeding. They can cause fluid retention and exacerbate any existing oedema and ascites.[8]

REFERENCES

1. Appendix 4: *Pregnancy*. British National Formulary; 55; 2008.

2. *Oral anticoagulants*. 2.8.2. British National Formulary; 55; 2008.

3. Appendix 3: *Renal impairment*. British National Formulary; 55; 2008

4. *Antipsychotic drugs*. 4.2.1. British National Formulary; 55; 2008.

5. Appendix 5: *Breast-feeding*. British National Formulary; 55; 2008.

6. *Gout and cytotoxic induced hyperuricaemia*. 10.1.4. British National Formulary; 55; 2008.

7. Driver and Vehicle Licensing Agency. *For Medical Practitioners: At a Glance Guide to the Current Medical Standards of Fitness to Drive.* February 2008 (cited 2008 April 29). Available from http://www.dvla.gov.uk/media/pdf/medical/aagv1.pdf

8. Appendix 2: *Liver disease*. British National Formulary; 55; 2008.

Chapter 9
Psychiatry and Neurology

QUESTIONS

THEME: SYMPTOMS OF PSYCHIATRIC DISORDERS

Options

A   Bipolar disorder
B   Borderline personality disorder
C   Depression
D   Dysthymia
E   Eating disorder
F   Generalised anxiety disorder
G   Obsessive-compulsive disorder
H   Panic disorder
I   Schizophrenia

For each of the symptoms below select the single psychiatric disorder from the list above of which it is most characteristic. Each option may be used once, more than once or not at all.

- [ ] **9.1 Agoraphobia**
- [ ] **9.2 Anhedonia**
- [ ] **9.3 Distorted body image**
- [ ] **9.4 Fear of abandonment**
- [ ] **9.5 Repeated hand washing**
- [ ] **9.6 Pressured speech**

THEME: DIAGNOSTIC AIDS IN PSYCHIATRY

Options

A   Alcohol addiction

B   Alzheimer disease

C   Anorexia nervosa

D   Borderline personality disorder

E   Depression

F   Generalised anxiety disorder

G   Postpartum depression

H   Post-traumatic stress disorder

I   Schizophrenia

J   Somatisation disorder

For each of the questionnaires below select the single psychiatric disorder from the list above in which it is most useful as an aid to diagnosis. Each option may be used once, more than once or not at all.

☐ **9.7**   **CAGE questionnaire**

☐ **9.8**   **Edinburgh (EPDS) Scale**

☐ **9.9**   **Mini-mental state examination (MMSE)**

☐ **9.10**   **Patient Health Questionnaire (PHQ 9)**

THEME: DRUG MANAGEMENT OF PSYCHIATRIC DISEASE

Options

A Amitriptyline

B Atropine

C Chlordiazepoxide

D Chlorpromazine

E Clozapine

F Citalopram

G Donepezil

H Haloperidol

I Lithium carbonate

J Lorazepam

K Olanzapine

For each of the patients below, select the single most appropriate drug that should be administered from the list of options above. Each option may be used once, more than once or not at all.

☐ **9.11** A 63-year-old man presents in an agitated state with confusion and visual hallucinations that terrify him. He has pyrexia, tremor and tachycardia and is sweating profusely. He has previously been seen with symptoms associated with chronic alcoholism.

☐ **9.12** A 30-year-old woman had presented in an agitated and distractible state. She had an expansive euphoric mood and would not stop talking. Her behaviour had recently resulted in dismissal from her job. After suitable anti-psychotic medication her symptoms have calmed. You note she has had previous similar episodes.

☐ **9.13** An 83-year old man gives a 3-month history of increasing insomnia, fatigue and difficulty concentrating. He has lost interest in daily activities and feels a burden on his family.

☐ **9.14** The police bring a 45-year-old man to casualty as he has been threatening staff at a nearby store. He has prominent third-person auditory hallucinations and states that the Queen of England, via a radiotransmitter implanted in his teeth, controls his actions.

☐ **9.15** A 68-year-old woman is brought in by her daughter, who feels she is becoming more forgetful. She scores 15 points on the mini-mental state examination. She is otherwise well.

THEME: DIAGNOSIS OF NEUROLOGICAL DISORDERS

Options

A   Bell's palsy
B   Carpal tunnel syndrome
C   Chorea
D   Diabetic neuropathy
E   Guillain–Barré syndrome
F   Motor neurone disease
G   Multiple sclerosis
H   Myaesthenia gravis
I   Restless legs syndrome
J   Syringomyelia

For each of the patients below select the single most likely neurological disorder from the list above. Each option may be used once, more than once or not at all.

☐ **9.16**   An 11-year-old girl is reported to have become increasingly clumsy, restless and emotional. She has uncoordinated jerking movements affecting the face, feet and hands.

☐ **9.17**   A 38-year-old man has felt unwell and had pain in the back for 4 days. His arms and legs have become weak and he is having difficulty going upstairs. There is also facial muscle weakness.

☐ **9.18**   A 65-year-old obese woman has had a burning feeling in her feet for 12 months and an ulcerated toe as though caused by an ill-fitting shoe. She was not aware of any trauma.

☐ **9.19**   A 60-year-old man complains of difficulty with vision because his upper lids droop over his eyes. He also has some double vision. He is worse in the evenings.

☐ **9.20** A 42-year-old woman has had muscle weakness, pins and needles and loss of sensation mainly in the lower limbs. The symptoms have been relapsing and remitting over 2 years. She also now has reduced vision.

☐ **9.21** A 55-year-old woman wakes in the early morning with pain and pins and needles in her hands.

THEME: HEADACHE

Options

A   Bacterial meningitis
B   Basilar migraine
C   Benign intracranial hypertension
D   Cerebrovascular accident
E   Chronic subdural haematoma
F   Cryptococcal meningitis
G   Herpes encephalitis
H   Normal-pressure hydrocephalus
I   Subarachnoid haemorrhage
J   Transient ischaemic attack

For each of the clinical scenarios below, which one of the list of options above would be the most appropriate cause of headache? Each option may be used once, more than once or not at all.

☐ **9.22**   A 75-year-old woman is brought into the surgery with a history of headache, forgetfulness and urinary incontinence for the preceding 3 weeks.

☐ **9.23**   A 23-year-old man has mild headache, low-grade fever and malaise. He has been unwell for 5 days. On examination you notice facial molluscum contagiosum.

☐ **9.24**   A 36-year-old man has sudden-onset of the worst headache he has ever experienced. The pain is mostly occipital and he has a reduced Glasgow Coma Scale score.

☐ **9.25**   A 19-year-old female university student has fever, headache and cervical rigidity.

☐ **9.26**   A 28-year-old rugby player presents to the surgery midway through the season with a 2-week history of headache, ataxia and difficulty passing urine.

☐ **9.27**   An obese 29-year-old woman presents with a 3-month history of recurrent headaches and associated visual disturbance. She takes an oral contraceptive and on examination she is noted to have papilloedema.

THEME: NEUROLOGICAL SYMPTOMS AND SIGNS

Options

A   Apraxia

B   Clonus

C   Cortical blindness

D   Dysarthria

E   Dyspraxia

F   Dysdiadochokinesis

G   Dysphasia

H   Fasciculation

I   Hemiparesis

J   Hemiplegia

K   Homonymous hemianopia

L   Past pointing

M   Romberg's sign

For each of the definitions below select the single neurological symptom or sign from the list above of which it is most characteristic. Each option may be used once, more than once or not at all.

☐ **9.28** Involuntary muscular contractions due to sudden stretching of the muscle

☐ **9.29** Impairment of speech and of comprehension of speech

☐ **9.30** Loss of vision at one side in both eyes

☐ **9.31** The partial loss of the ability to coordinate and perform certain purposeful movements and gestures in the absence of motor or sensory impairments

☐ **9.32** The partial paralysis of one side of the body

☐ **9.33** The patient falls when the eyes are closed

☐ **9.34** An inability to perform rapid, alternating movements

9.35   A 40-year-old woman has been receiving fluoxetine 20mg daily for 6 weeks for an episode of major depression. She is feeling much better and wants to stop the drug.

Select from the list below the single most appropriate management option.

- [ ] **A**   Agree and stop the drug immediately
- [ ] **B**   Recommend that she needs to take the same dose for at least 6 months more
- [ ] **C**   Suggest that the same dose should be taken indefinitely to prevent relapse
- [ ] **D**   Suggest that she wean off slowly over the next month
- [ ] **E**   Stop the drug and refer for cognitive behaviour therapy

9.36   A 58-year-old woman has headaches, dizziness, palpitations, chest discomfort, excessive sweating, nausea, nervousness, difficulty sleeping, poor concentration, muscle and joint pains in the arms and numbness and paraesthesias in the fingers on both hands. Symptoms have worsened over 12 months. Physical examination, thyroid function and ECG are normal. She appears anxious and takes deep sighing breaths periodically. This is her first presentation with these symptoms.

Select from the list below the single most likely diagnosis.

- [ ] **A**   Depression
- [ ] **B**   Generalised anxiety disorder
- [ ] **C**   Panic disorder
- [ ] **D**   Post-traumatic stress disorder
- [ ] **E**   Somatisation disorder

9.37   A 24-year-old woman presents with a sudden-onset, severe headache with retro-orbital pain and photophobia, associated with two episodes of vomiting. She says it is the worst headache she has ever had. There is no past history of migraine. Examination reveals no neurological deficit.

What is the single most appropriate initial investigation from the list below?

☐ **A**   Computed tomography (CT) scan of the head

☐ **B**   Erythrocyte sedimentation rate (ESR)

☐ **C**   Lumbar puncture

☐ **D**   Magnetic resonance imaging (MRI) of the head

☐ **E**   Technetium brain scan

9.38   A 46-year-old woman has persistent morning headaches and vomiting. A CT scan shows a space-occupying lesion in the temporal lobe. Assessment of her visual fields reveals a defect.

What is the single most likely defect from the options below?

☐ **A**   Bitemporal hemianopia

☐ **B**   Homonymous hemianopia

☐ **C**   Homonymous lower quadrantic defect

☐ **D**   Homonymous upper quadrantic defect

☐ **E**   Unilateral visual loss

9.39   **A 65-year-old man presents with slowness, stiffness, tremor and loss of balance. You suspect Parkinson's disease.**

Select from the list below the single true statement regarding the management of this condition.

☐   A   Early use of medication is indicated

☐   B   Initial high dose of levodopa is beneficial

☐   C   Old age does not cause such symptoms

☐   D   Patients must inform the Driver and Vehicle Licensing Agency (DVLA)

☐   E   Polypharmacy is to be avoided

ANSWERS

THEME: SYMPTOMS OF PSYCHIATRIC DISORDERS

9.1   H   Panic disorder

Agoraphobia is an anxiety disorder, often precipitated by the fear of having a panic attack in a place from which there is no easy means of escape. As a result, sufferers may avoid public or unfamiliar places. Triggers may include crowds, wide open spaces or travelling, even for short distances. The anxiety is made worse by a fear of social embarrassment, as the agoraphobic fears a panic attack and appearing distressed in public. If severe, the sufferer may become confined to the home (their personal safety zone).

9.2   C   Depression

Anhedonia is an inability to experience enjoyment from normally pleasurable life events such as eating, exercise, and social interaction. Anhedonia is recognised as one of the important symptoms of depression. It is also seen in schizophrenia.

9.3   E   Anorexia nervosa

A distorted body image and fear of becoming overweight are features of anorexia nervosa. The origin of this is complex. The media sets an unrealistic standard of beauty that makes many people feel inadequate and dissatisfied and forces them to strive for an unattainable appearance. In addition a critical and unaffectionate upbringing can lead to poor self-esteem. Other environmental stresses, including sexual, physical, and emotional abuse, racism, and poverty may also be important. Women from deprived or racial minorities find they are forced to live in a culture that has a narrowly-defined conception of beauty.

9.4   B   Borderline personality disorder

Borderline personality disorder (BPD) is a serious mental illness characterised by pervasive instability in moods, interpersonal relationships, self-image, and behaviour. This instability often disrupts family and work life, long-term planning, and the sense of self-identity. It was once thought to be a psychosis. In fact people with BPD suffer from a disorder of emotion regulation. While less well known than schizophrenia or bipolar disorder, BPD is more common. Sufferers often have highly unstable social relationships. While they can develop intense but stormy attachments, their attitudes towards family, friends, and loved ones may suddenly change from admiration and love to anger and dislike. Even with family members, people with BPD are highly sensitive to rejection, reacting with anger and distress even to such mild separations such as an absence on a holiday. In such situations the individual with BPD feels lost and worthless. Suicide threats and attempts may occur due to the anger at perceived abandonment. There is also a high rate of self-injury without suicide intent.

9.5   G   Obsessive-compulsive disorder

Obsessive-compulsive disorder (OCD) is an anxiety disorder characterised by a person's obsessive, distressing, intrusive thoughts and related compulsions (tasks or rituals) which attempt to neutralise the obsessions. Typical symptoms are the need to check things repeatedly or washing hands over and over again.

9.6   A   Bipolar disorder

Bipolar disorder is characterised by episodes of abnormally elevated mood, clinically referred to as mania. Individuals who experience manic episodes also commonly experience depressive episodes, or mixed episodes in which features of both mania and depression are present. Pressure of speech is a characteristic symptom of mania. There is a tendency to speak rapidly, as if motivated by urgency not apparent to the listener. The speech produced is difficult to interrupt and may be too fast for the listener to understand. People with schizophrenia, as well as anyone experiencing extreme anxiety, may also exhibit pressure of speech.

THEME: DIAGNOSTIC AIDS IN PSYCHIATRY

9.7   A   Alcohol addiction

This is a screening questionnaire devised to identify problematic drinking in an outpatient department or primary care setting. It comprises a four item questionnaire about: **C**utting down drinking; **A**nnoyed by criticism; **G**uilty about drinking; **E**ye-opener drink – needing a drink first thing in the morning. Positive answers to two or more questions are indicative of problem drinking.

9.8   G   Postpartum depression

The Edinburgh post-natal depression scale[1, 2] is a 10-item self-reporting questionnaire used to screen for postnatal depression.

9.9   B   Alzheimer disease

The Mini-Mental state examination is a 30-item objective assessment test that can be used to screen for Alzheimer disease (AD) as well as to monitor prognosis. A score below 26 is usually indicative of mild AD. Recent National Institute for Health and Clinical excellence (NICE) guidelines recommend the prescription of anti-dementia medication for patients with MMSE scores between 20 and 10.[3] It tests orientation for time and place, the ability to repeat the names of three objects, the ability to subtract 7 from 100 (serial 7s), the ability to recall the names of the three objects, tests of language, writing a sentence and the ability to follow commands and finally the ability to copy a simple drawing.

9.10   E   Depression

All new diagnoses of depression should have an assessment of severity, on which to base management decisions and monitor progress. Several questionnaires have been recommended for this purpose including the Patient Health Questionnaire (PHQ-9) (Table 1).[4]

Table 1: Questions asked in PHQ-9

Over the last two weeks, how often have you been bothered by any of the following problems?

- Little interest or pleasure in doing things?
- Feeling down, depressed, or hopeless?
- Trouble falling or staying asleep, or sleeping too much?
- Feeling tired or having little energy?
- Poor appetite or overeating?
- Feeling bad about yourself – or that you are a failure or have let yourself or your family down?
- Trouble concentrating on things, such as reading the newspaper or watching television?
- Moving or speaking so slowly that other people could have noticed? Or the opposite – being so fidgety or restless that you have been moving around a lot more than usual?
- Thoughts that you would be better off dead, or of hurting yourself in some way?

For each question the response can be

- Not at all
- Several days (score 1)
- More than half the days (score 2)
- Nearly every day (score 3)

Depression Severity: 0-4 None, 5-9 Mild depression, 10-14 Moderate depression, 15-19 Moderately severe depression, 20-27 Severe depression.

THEME: DRUG MANAGEMENT OF PSYCHIATRIC DISEASE

9.11   C   Chlordiazepoxide

Delirium tremens typically presents acutely after 3–4 days of abstinence from alcohol. When fully developed the syndrome includes vivid visual hallucinations (not definitely required for the diagnosis), delusions, confusion, agitation and autonomic arousal (often including pyrexia). While short lived (a few days), mortality can be up to 20%. Treatment is fluid replacement and sedation with diazepam or chlordiazepoxide with close monitoring for electrolyte imbalance (especially hypokalaemia).

9.12   I   Lithium carbonate

Bipolar disorders consist of marked changes in mood that vary from major depressive episodes to major manic episodes. A manic episode consists of a sustained period (at least a week) when mood is abnormally and persistently elevated, expansive or irritable. Symptoms include inflated self-esteem (which may be delusional), decreased need for sleep, talkativeness, flight of ideas, distractibility; they typically cause marked impairment in occupational functioning or relationships with others. The average age of onset of bipolar disorder is about 30 years. Treatment of the acute manic phase is often in hospital.

Treatment of the agitation in acute manic episodes requires the use of antipsychotic medications, such as quetiapine, olanzapine and chlorpromazine. The mainstay of treatment is a mood stabiliser medication. These comprise several unrelated compounds which have been shown to be effective in preventing relapses of mania. The gold standard mood stabiliser is lithium, while almost as widely used is sodium valproate, originally used as an anticonvulsant. Other anticonvulsants used in bipolar disorder include carbamazepine and lamotrigine.

CHAPTER 9 ANSWERS

9.13   F   Citalopram

Symptoms of depression are the commonest psychiatric symptoms in community samples of elderly adults. As with all depressive symptoms, when symptoms become more marked, particularly when disturbing sleep or appetite, then antidepressant medications should be used. In patients who present primarily with insomnia (or agitation), amitriptyline is sometimes used for its sedating effects, particularly given at bedtime. However, tricyclics are associated with arrhythmias and should be avoided in the elderly or patients with cardiovascular disease. The tricyclics are also more dangerous in overdose, so suicide risk should be frequently assessed. The most likely first choice in this scenario would be citalopram, as it is a serotonin selective reuptake inhibitor (SSRI) with sedative properties. The SSRIs have a much better safety profile in this age group.

9.14   K   Olanzapine

Schizophrenia is characterised by psychotic symptoms during the active phase of the illness. Symptoms include bizarre delusions (eg involving a phenomenon that the individual's culture would regard as totally implausible such as thoughts being broadcast out loud), prominent hallucinations (often a voice commenting on the individual's behaviour or thoughts), incoherent speech, catatonic behaviour and flat or inappropriate affect. During the course of the illness, there is significant deterioration in social functioning and self-care. The goal of treatment initially is to decrease symptom occurrence. Medication dosage is increased as long as hallucinations, delusions and disorganised thinking continue; the most frequent limiting factor is the appearance of extrapyramidal side-effects.

Though expensive, the newer atypical antipsychotic drugs are usually preferred for initial treatment over the older typical antipsychotics. They are often better tolerated and associated with lower rates of tardive dyskinesia, although they are more likely to induce weight gain and obesity-related diseases. Treatment-resistant schizophrenia is a term used for the failure of symptoms to respond satisfactorily to at least two different antipsychotics. Patients in this category may be prescribed clozapine.[5]

9.15 G Donepezil

Anticholinesterase inhibiting drugs (donepezil, galantamine and rivastigmine) are recommended for the adjunctive treatment of moderate Alzheimer disease in those whose mini-mental state score (MMSE) is 10–20 points. Up to half of patients given these drugs will show a slower rate of cognitive decline. Patients must attend a specialist clinic where in addition to MMSE score the clinic should assess cognitive, global and behavioural functioning, activities of daily living, and the likelihood of compliance with treatment. Care can be continued by general practitioners under a shared-care protocol. It can be continued until patients, carers or specialists think it appropriate to stop.[3]

THEME: DIAGNOSIS OF NEUROLOGICAL DISORDERS

9.16 C Chorea

Sydenham's chorea is also known as 'Saint Vitus Dance'. It results from childhood infection with Group A β-hemolytic streptococci. It may occur up to 6 months after the acute infection and may occasionally be the presenting symptom of rheumatic fever. It is more common in females and most patients are under 18 years. Typically the onset of chorea is acute, usually affecting all limbs. Other motor symptoms include facial grimacing, hypotonia, loss of fine motor control and a gait disturbance. Half of patients spontaneously recover after 2–6 months whilst mild or moderate chorea or other motor symptoms can persist for as long as 2 years or more. Sydenham's is also associated with psychiatric symptoms, with obsessive-compulsive disorder being the most frequent symptom. Movements cease during sleep.

9.17 E Guillain-Barré syndrome

Guillain-Barré syndrome (GBS) is usually preceded by an acute infection triggering an autoimmune attack on peripheral nerves. It is characterised by weakness of the lower limbs first, rapidly progressing in an ascending fashion, usually over periods of hours or days, the arms and facial muscles also becoming affected. Frequently, the lower cranial nerves may be involved, leading to bulbar weakness causing difficulty with swallowing, drooling, and maintaining an open airway and respiratory difficulties. Most patients need to be in hospital and may require ventilatory assistance. Sensory loss, if present, usually involves loss of proprioception and complete loss of deep tendon reflexes. Loss of pain and temperature sensation is usually mild. Pain is in fact a common symptom in GBS, presenting as deep aching pain usually in the weakened muscles. Bladder dysfunction may occur in severe cases.

9.18 D Diabetic neuropathy

This woman has diabetes leading to a sensorimotor neuropathy. Longer nerve fibres are affected more than shorter ones, because nerve conduction velocity is slowed in proportion to a nerve's length. Decreased sensation and loss of reflexes occurs first in the toes, and then extends upward. There is a glove-stocking distribution of numbness, sensory loss, distortion of sensation and night-time pain. The pain can feel like burning, or a pricking sensation, or an ache. Pins and needles are common. Proprioception is affected early. These patients cannot feel when they are stepping on a splinter or when a shoe is ill-fitting. Consequently, they are at risk for ulcers and infections on the feet and legs. Similarly, they can get fractures and develop a Charcot joint. Loss of motor function results in dorsiflexion, contractures of the toes with loss of the inter-osseous muscle function and contraction of the digits (hammer toes). These contractures may also occur in the hand. The condition is progressive.

9.19   H   Myasthenia gravis

Myasthenia gravis is an autoimmune neuromuscular disorder leading to muscle weakness that increases during activity. Muscles that control eye and eyelid movement, facial expression, chewing, talking, and swallowing are most likely to be involved. The muscles of respiration and neck and limb movements can also be affected. Often the physical examination is normal. In most cases, the first noticeable symptom is weakness of the eye muscles (asymmetrical ptosis, diplopia). Other symptoms may be unstable or waddling gait; weakness in arms, hands, fingers, legs, and neck; a change in facial expression; dysphagia; shortness of breath, and dysarthria. In some, difficulty in swallowing and slurred speech may be the first signs. The circulating antibodies in myasthenia gravis block acetylcholine receptors. Myasthenia is treated medically with cholinesterase inhibitors or immunosuppressants, and, in some, thymectomy. It is an uncommon disease.

9.20   G   Multiple sclerosis

Multiple sclerosis (MS) is an autoimmune condition, leading to nerve demyelination. MS takes several forms, with new symptoms occurring either in discrete attacks (relapsing forms) or slowly progressing over time (progressive forms). Symptoms may include reduced sensation, muscle weakness, abnormal muscle spasms, or difficulty in moving, difficulties with coordination and balance (ataxia), dysarthria or dysphagia, visual problems (nystagmus, optic neuritis, reduced visual acuity or diplopia), fatigue and acute or chronic pain syndromes, and bladder and bowel difficulties. Cognitive impairment or emotional symptomatology is also common. Neuropathic pain is usual and distressing. The pain usually occurs in the legs and may be accompanied by paraesthesia. The initial attacks of multiple sclerosis are often transient, mild and self-limited. They often do not prompt a consultation and sometimes are only identified in retrospect after the diagnosis has been made. The most common initial symptoms reported are changes in sensation in the arms, legs or face, complete or partial vision loss (optic neuritis), weakness, double vision or unsteadiness when walking.

9.21   B   Carpal tunnel syndrome

Carpal tunnel syndrome is a condition in which the median nerve is compressed in the carpal tunnel at the wrist. Many people with carpal tunnel syndrome have gradually increasing symptoms over time. The first symptoms typically include numbness and burning and tingling in the fingers, usually the thumb, index, and middle fingers. Symptoms appear in the early morning because many people sleep with bent wrists further compressing the carpal tunnel. Difficulty gripping, dropping objects, and weakness suggest progression. Later there may be wasting of the thenar muscles. In early stages patients often mistakenly blame the symptoms on restricted circulation and believe their hands are simply falling asleep. In most cases of CTS a cause is not obvious. A common factor in developing symptoms is increased hand use or activity.

THEME: HEADACHE

9.22   H   Normal-pressure hydrocephalus

This is usually a disorder of the elderly. There is enlargement of the cerebral ventricles without an increase in the cerebrospinal fluid pressure. It commonly presents with dementia, ataxia and urinary incontinence.

9.23   F   Cryptococcal meningitis

This is an acquired immune deficiency syndrome (AIDS)-defining illness. It occurs in patients with a low CD4 count. It often has a slowly evolving prodromal phase with fever, malaise and headache. Patients may have nausea, vomiting and photophobia and neck stiffness at the time of presentation. Indian-ink staining of the cerebrospinal fluid shows *Cryptococcus neoformans*. Treatment is with the intravenous antifungal agents amphotericin and/or flucytosine. Facial molluscum contagiosum is a good indicator of immunosuppression in HIV infection.

9.24   I   Subarachnoid haemorrhage

This patient has had a spontaneous bleed into the subarachnoid space. It classically presents with very severe headache of sudden onset. The initial pain is often in the occipital region. Patients may remain well or be very seriously ill on presentation. Diagnosis is by CT scan or lumbar puncture if the CT scan is negative and no focal lesion is demonstrated. It is often associated with underlying saccular (berry) aneurysms or arteriovenous (AV) malformations.

9.25   A   Bacterial meningitis

This girl has bacterial meningitis. She has the classic signs of fever, headache and neck stiffness. Photophobia and vomiting are often present. Meningococcal (*Neisseria meningitidis*) meningitis should be immediately suspected. There may or may not be a petechial rash. Cefotaxime/ceftriaxone therapy should be commenced as soon as possible if meningococcal meningitis is thought likely. This disease may show rapid progression from being fully well to septicaemia and the value of early antibiotics should not be underestimated. Lumbar puncture should be avoided.

9.26   E   Chronic subdural haematoma

This is caused by slow bleeding from a vein into the subdural space. Gradually symptoms result from haematoma accumulation over a period of days or weeks. There may be headache, reduced mental capacity or more focal signs. Elderly people and alcohol misusers are at highest risk but trauma can be a cause in any age group.

9.27   C   Benign intracranial hypertension

This uncommon disorder often occurs in overweight women. It represents an increase in cerebrospinal fluid pressure without an increase in the size of the cerebral ventricles. It causes headache and visual blurring due to papilloedema. It may be associated with steroids and tetracycline treatment. Thiazide diuretics and acetazolamide may be useful in management. Weight reduction may also be helpful.

THEME: NEUROLOGICAL SYMPTOMS AND SIGNS

9.28   C   Clonus

Clonus is particularly associated with upper motor neuron lesions such as amyotrophic lateral sclerosis, stroke, multiple sclerosis, spinal cord damage and hepatic encephalopathy. Unlike the small, spontaneous twitching known as fasciculations (usually benign but can be caused by lower motor neuron pathology as in motor neurone disease), clonus causes larger muscle action.

9.29   G   Dysphasia

It is caused by brain damage, usually in the left side of the brain which is responsible for language and communication. The term aphasia is sometimes used instead. Aphasia literally means no speech but the impairment in aphasia may range from complete absence of speech to difficulty in naming objects. Dysarthria is a motor speech disorder resulting from neurological injury, characterised by poor articulation (cf dysphasia: disorder of the content of speech).

9.30   K   Homonymous hemianopia

The neurological damage to the optic tracts has occurred behind the optic chiasma. Cortical blindness is the total or partial loss of vision in a normal-appearing eye caused by damage to the visual area in the occipital cortex.

9.31   E   Dyspraxia

Dyspraxia may be acquired (eg as a result of brain damage due to stroke or other trauma), or associated with failure or delay of normal neurological development (developmental dyspraxia). The term apraxia is more often used to describe this symptom, although apraxia strictly denotes a complete (as opposed to partial) loss of a particular function.

9.32   I   Hemiparesis

It is caused by lesions of the corticospinal tract, which runs from the cortex of the frontal lobe to the motor neurons of the spinal cord and is responsible for the movements of the muscles of the body and limbs. The tract passes through the midbrain, pons and medulla, respectively. It crosses to the opposite side on the lowest portion of the medulla and goes down the opposite side of the spinal cord to meet the contralateral motor neurons. Hence, one side of the brain controls muscle movements of the opposite side of the body, and thus the disruption of the right corticospinal tract in the brain stem or upper brain causes a hemiparesis on the left side of the body and vice versa. On the other hand, the lesions of the tract occurring in the spinal cord lead to a hemiparesis on the same side of the body. The facial muscles are also controlled by the same tract. Hemiplegia involves a complete paralysis of one half of a patient's body

9.33   M   Romberg's sign

Romberg's test is used to assess the dorsal columns of the spinal cord. These are essential for joint position sense (proprioception). A positive test suggests that ataxia is sensory in nature, ie depending on loss of proprioception. A negative test suggests that it is cerebellar, ie depending on cerebellar dysfunction instead. Romberg's test is positive in conditions that affect the dorsal columns of the spinal cord, such as tabes dorsalis (neurosyphilis) and conditions affecting the sensory nerves (sensory peripheral neuropathies), such as chronic inflammatory demyelinating polyradiculoneuropathy. Past pointing is pointing beyond the finger in the finger–nose test and demonstrates an inability to coordinate fine motor activities (intention tremor). It is a sign of cerebellar dysfunction.

9.34   F   Dysdiadochokinesis

Dysdiadochokinesis is also a sign of cerebellar dysfunction. An example is the inability to rapidly flip the hands.

9.35   B   Recommend that she needs to take the same dose for at least 6 months more

Pharmacologic treatment for major depression should last for a minimum of 6 months after an initial episode. Most clinicians will continue treatment for at least 1 year for patients with a second episode or for patients over 60 years. If the patient has responded, and symptoms are resolved, the decision can be made whether to taper the patient off the drug or continue maintenance therapy. Many patients relapse after cessation of therapy. Antidepressant drugs are not usually effective for mild depression and cognitive behaviour therapy should be considered initially.

9.36   B   Generalised anxiety disorder

The diagnosis requires excessive anxiety and worry for most days over 6 months and inability to control the worry. The anxiety will involve a variety of events or activities. Other symptoms may include restlessness or feeling keyed up or on edge, fatigue, irritability, muscle tension, difficulty falling or staying asleep and difficulty concentrating or the mind going blank. Patients with a diagnosed anxiety disorder also have high rates of co-morbid depression. Some patients can be regarded as having mixed anxiety-depressive disorder, and they have a significantly increased risk of developing full-blown depression or anxiety. Somatisation disorder (hysteria) is a diagnosis applied to patients who chronically and persistently complain of varied physical symptoms that have no identifiable physical origin. Post-traumatic stress disorder is an anxiety disorder that can develop after exposure to one or more terrifying events in which serious physical harm occurred or was threatened.

9.37   D   Patients must inform the Driver and Vehicle Licensing Agency (DVLA)[6]

It can be very difficult sometimes to distinguish parkinsonian symptoms from the natural features of old age. There is rarely any urgency to prescribe and patients should be referred for specialist assessment to establish the diagnosis and initiate management. Levodopa works but after 4–5 years it becomes less effective with dyskinesias and fluctuations developing. Lower doses are less likely to be associated with these long-term problems. Polypharmacy becomes inevitable over time as drugs are added to enhance the effect of levodopa (eg entacapone, bromocriptine, cabergoline).[7]

9.38   A   CT scan of the head

CT imaging is the initial investigation of choice, which usually shows the presence of subarachnoid or intraventricular blood. A lumbar puncture is unnecessary if a subarachnoid haemorrhage is confirmed by CT, but should be considered if doubt remains. The CSF becomes yellow (xanthochromic) about 12 hours after a subarachnoid haemorrhage. MR angiography is usually performed in all patients who are potentially fit for surgery.

9.39   D   Homonymous upper quadrantic defect

Temporal lobe lesions cause an upper quadrantic defect and parietal lobes a lower one. A lesion to the optic chiasma causes bitemporal hemianopia. Optic tract lesions cause field defects, which are homonymous, hemianopic and often incomplete and incongruous.

CHAPTER 9 ANSWERS

REFERENCES

1. Cox JL, Holden JM and Sagovosky R. Detection of Postnatal Depression. Development of the 10-item Edinburgh Postnatal Depression Scale. Br J Psychiatry 1987 150: 782-6.

2. Murray L, Carothers AD. The validation of the Edinburgh Post-natal Depression Scale on a community sample. Br J Psychiatry 1990 157: 288-90.

3. National Institute for Health and Clinical Excellence. *Alzheimer's disease – donepezil, galantamine, rivastigmine (review) and memantine* (homepage on the Internet), September 2007 (cited 2008 April 30). Available from http://www.nice.org.uk/TA111

4. Kroenke K, Spitzer RL, Williams JB. The PHQ-9: Validity of a brief depression severity measure. *J Gen Intern Med.* 2001 Sep;16(9): 606-13.

5. National Institute for Health and Clinical Excellence. *Schizophrenia – atypical antipsychotics* (homepage on the Internet), June 2002 (cited 2008 April 30). Available from http://www.nice.org.uk/guidance/index.jsp?action=byID&o=11460

6. Driver and Vehicle Licensing Agency. *For Medical Practitioners: At a glance Guide to the current Medical Standards of Fitness to Drive.* February 2008 (cited 2008 April 29). Available from http://www.dvla.gov.uk/media/pdf/medical/aagv1.pdf

7. The Primary Care Task Force for the Parkinson's Disease Society. *Parkinson's aware in primary care.* (homepage on the Internet), September 2003 (cited 2008 May 1). Available from http://www.parkinsons.org.uk/pdf/PDAwarePrimaryCareSept03.pdf

Chapter 10
Renal and Urology

QUESTIONS

THEME: LOW URINE OUTPUT AFTER SURGERY

Options

A Acute interstitial nephritis
B Acute urinary retention
C Blocked catheter
D Chronic kidney disease
E Renal hypoperfusion due to hypotension
F Renal hypoperfusion due to intravascular depletion
G Urinary infection

For each of the following presentations, choose the most likely cause from the list of options above. Each option may be used once, more than once or not at all.

☐ **10.1** An 80-year-old man is usually hypertensive. He is postoperative day 1 following hemicolectomy. He has epidural analgesia for the pain. His urine output reduces after he is given his usual long-term medication.

☐ **10.2** A 65-year-old man has undergone hernia repair as a day case. He has not passed urine since the procedure, and on examination there is a suprapubic mass.

☐ **10.3** A 73-year-old man has undergone a transurethral resection of the prostate (TURP). In spite of irrigation his urine is heavily blood stained and he is passing < 20ml/h of urine.

☐ **10.4** A 35-year-old man has had a subtotal colectomy for ulcerative colitis. He has been given gentamicin as prophylaxis and diclofenac for analgesia. On the first postoperative day his urine output has tailed off to < 10ml/h.

THEME: INVESTIGATIONS FOR RENAL DISEASES

Options

A   Antegrade pyelography
B   Computed tomography (CT) scan
C   Dipstick urinalysis
D   Micturating cystography
E   Magnetic resonance imaging (MRI)
F   Plain X-ray
G   Renal arteriography
H   Renal biopsy
I   Renal scintigraphy
J   Retrograde pyelography
K   Ultrasound scan

For each of the case scenarios below, choose the most appropriate investigation from the list of options above. Each option may be used once, more than once or not at all.

☐ **10.5** This investigation would be needed to diagnose the problem in a patient who had rising urea and creatinine levels after taking an angiotensin-converting enzyme (ACE) inhibitor for a couple of weeks.

☐ **10.6** This is a useful investigation for recurrent urinary tract infection, especially in adults with disturbed bladder function. It can be combined with urodynamic measurements of bladder pressure and urethral flow.

☐ **10.7** A useful investigation for patients with suspected ureteric colic who have no stones visible on ultrasound or plain abdominal X-ray.

☐ **10.8** This is the investigation of choice for diagnosing polycystic kidney disease, measuring renal size and detecting renal vein thrombosis.

THEME: DIAGNOSIS OF RENAL DISEASE

Options

A Acute tubulointerstitial nephritis
B Analgesic nephropathy
C Contrast medium-induced nephropathy
D Haemolytic uraemic syndrome
E Idiopathic thrombocytopenic purpura
F IgA nephropathy
G Medullary cystic kidney disease
H Retroperitoneal fibrosis
I Streptococcal glomerulonephritis

For each of the patients below, choose the most likely diagnosis from the list of options above. Each option may be used once, more than once or not at all.

☐ **10.9** A 10-year-old boy has had a sore throat, which he thinks he caught from his friend who returned from Africa last week. His parents think his limbs are starting to swell, and this morning he told them his urine was red. On bedside urine testing there is blood and protein in his urine.

☐ **10.10** A 48-year-old woman has noticed recent ankle swelling, a feeling of abdominal bloating, and she thinks she is passing less urine than usual. She recently had a CT scan.

☐ **10.11** A 5-year-old girl experiences an episode of severe diarrhoea following a recent school trip to a farm. She now has haematuria and her blood results show thrombocytopenia and her urea and electrolytes are rising.

☐ **10.12** A 62-year-old man with a previous history of surgery for abdominal aortic aneurysm presented with malaise, backache and normochromic anaemia, uraemia and a raised erythrocyte sedimentation rate (ESR). A peri-aortic mass is seen on CT.

THEME: MANAGEMENT OF ACUTE RENAL FAILURE

Options

A   Angiotensin-converting enzyme (ACE) inhibitor

B   Calcium resonium orally/per rectum

C   Catheterisation

D   Continuous ambulatory peritoneal dialysis (CAPD)

E   Haemodilution

F   Haemofiltration

G   Intravenous calcium gluconate

H   Insulin plus dextrose

I   Intravenous fluid

J   Intravenous furosemide

For each of the patients below, choose the most appropriate management option from the list above. Each option may be used once, more than once or not at all.

☐ **10.13** A 64-year-old man with end-stage renal disease, limited exercise tolerance due to chronic obstructive pulmonary disease and a colostomy due to a past history of ulcerative colitis has acute deterioration in his renal function.

☐ **10.14** An 85-year-old man presents with anuria for the past 72 hours. He is confused and restless. Examination reveals a distended lower abdomen and bi-basal chest crepitations. His potassium is 5.8mmol/l, urea 40mmol/l and creatinine 760μmol/l.

10.15 A 42-year-old previously fit and healthy man presents with a traumatic fractured neck of femur. A large haematoma is drained during surgery. Since the operation he has had episodes of vomiting and complains of thirst and malaise. His blood tests reveal sodium 152mmol/l, potassium 3.4mmol/l, urea 26mmol/l and creatinine 176μmol/l.

Normal values

- Sodium (Na): 135–145mmol/l
- Potassium (K): 3.5–5.0mmol/l
- Urea (Ur): 2.5–6.7mmol/l
- Creatinine (Cr): 70–< 150μmol/l

10.16 A 62-year-old man with severe cardiovascular disease is taking perindopril, furosemide, spironolactone and carvedilol for heart failure. His potassium level has been slowly rising and has been 6.5mmol/l for the past few weeks. The cardiologists are reluctant to change his heart failure medications as this regimen seems to have optimised his cardiac function. However, they wish to deal with his potassium level before it goes any higher. He is asymptomatic with no changes on electrocardiography.

CHAPTER 10 QUESTIONS

THEME: MANAGEMENT OF CHRONIC KIDNEY DISEASE

Options

A   Angiotensin-converting enzyme (ACE) inhibitor

B   β-Blocker

C   Calcium/cholecalciferol supplements

D   Erythropoiesis-stimulating agents

E   Giovannetti diet

F   Granulocyte colony-stimulating factor

G   Oral phosphodiesterase inhibitor

H   Pneumococcal vaccine

For each of the patients below, choose the most appropriate management option from the list of options above. Each option may be used once, more than once or not at all.

☐ **10.17   A 60-year-old man is diagnosed as having stage 3 chronic kidney disease (CKD). His parathormone (PTH) level is raised and 25-hydroxyvitamin D level is low.**

☐ **10.18   A 72-year-old man has routine monitoring of haemoglobin, potassium, calcium and phosphate for stage 3 CKD. His haemoglobin is found to be 9.0g/l (normal 13.5–18g/l). Investigations for occult bleeding are negative. He is getting too breathless to walk upstairs, and has started sleeping downstairs.**

☐ **10.19   A 78-year-old woman has just been diagnosed with stage 3 CKD. Her medications include alendronate, Calcichew D3 (calcium salt), lisinopril and omeprazole. She does not have any symptoms at present.**

☐ **10.20   A 65-year-old man receiving continuous ambulatory peritoneal dialysis (CAPD) for hypertensive nephropathy complains of distressing impotence. There is no history of coronary artery disease.**

THEME: INCONTINENCE

Options

A Anticholinergics

B Bladder training

C Catheter

D Colposuspension operation

E Cystoscopy

F Frequency/volume chart

G Midstream sample of urine

H Pad collection of urine

I Pelvic floor exercises

For each clinical scenario below, choose the most appropriate next step in management from the list of options above. Each option may be used once, more than once or not at all.

☐ **10.21** A 23-year-old woman presents with a 3-day history of frequency and dysuria. A couple of times she waited too long to pass urine and found she did not quite make it to the toilet before suddenly losing control.

☐ **10.22** A 38-year-old woman had her third baby by vaginal delivery 6 months ago. She complains of leaking small amounts of urine whenever she coughs or sneezes.

☐ **10.23** An 80-year-old man has been complaining of longstanding constipation. After many months of laxatives this seems to be improving, but during this time he has developed urinary incontinence. He tells you he passes urine every half an hour during the day, and is getting up several times in the night. He is being treated for benign prostatic hypertrophy and now has a good urinary flow.

☐ **10.24** A 75-year-old woman complains of needing to wear a pad day and night due to urinary incontinence. It happens without warning but more so if she strains or bends down. She has tried pelvic floor exercises for more than 3 months, and is intolerant of medication.

THEME: PENILE AND SCROTAL LUMPS

Options

A Epidermal cyst

B Epididymal cyst

C Epididymo-orchitis

D Haematoma

E Hernia

F Hydrocele

G Spermatocele

H Sperm granuloma

I Testicular cancer

J Torsion of the testis

K Varicocele

For each patient below select the single most likely diagnosis from the list above. Each option may be selected once, more than once or not at all.

☐ **10.25** A 55-year-old man has a firm, smooth, slightly tender lump, 1cm across above, behind and separate from the right testicle.

☐ **10.26** A 36-year-old man complains of testicular discomfort and a lump. The lower half of the right testicle is tender, swollen and hard.

☐ **10.27** A 14-year-old boy rapidly develops left scrotal pain and vomiting. The testis is enlarged tender and hard.

☐ **10.28** A 32-year-old man has a swollen left hemi-scrotum 2 days post vasectomy. His temperature is normal, the scrotum is tender and it is not possible to feel the testicle. There is some bruising of the skin around the incision site.

☐ **10.29** A 40-year-old man has a chronic ache in the right side of the scrotum with a small tender nodule that is separate from the testicle. He has previously had a vasectomy.

10.30 A 56-year-old man has been treated for many years with felodipine for hypertension. Now this is not adequately controlling his blood pressure, and angiotensin-converting enzyme (ACE) inhibitor treatment is planned. On routine baseline blood tests prior to commencing treatment the estimated glomerular filtration rate (eGFR) is 49ml/min/ 1.73m² (normal > 90ml/min/1.73m²).

From the following list of options choose the single most appropriate next step in his management.

- [ ] **A** Commence the ACE inhibitor as planned
- [ ] **B** Examine the patient, and do urinalysis
- [ ] **C** Recheck blood tests in 2 weeks
- [ ] **D** Refer him to the on-call medic for immediate admission
- [ ] **E** Refer to the local nephrology outpatients

10.31 A 60-year-old man complains of hesitancy and poor urinary stream. He has an enlarged benign prostate on examination. He has an international prostate symptom score (I-PSS) of 14 on a scale of 0–35 (moderately severe symptoms).

Select from the list below the single most appropriate management option.

- [ ] **A** Finasteride
- [ ] **B** Finasteride plus tamsulosin
- [ ] **C** Tamsulosin
- [ ] **D** Transurethral resection of prostate
- [ ] **E** Watchful waiting

10.32   A 19-year-old man is worried about the appearance of his penis and thinks he may have a sexually transmitted disease. He has diffuse small, painless, raised, white spots 1–3mm in diameter on the shaft of the penis that are more prominent when the skin is stretched.

Select from the list below the single most likely diagnosis.

- [ ] **A**   Fordyce's spots
- [ ] **B**   Penile warts
- [ ] **C**   Peyronie's disease
- [ ] **D**   Scabetic nodules
- [ ] **E**   Syphilis

10.33   The parents of a 2-year-old boy complain that the end of his penis 'balloons' when he passes urine. They ask if he needs circumcision. On gentle examination you are unable to retract his foreskin.

Select from the list below the single most likely diagnosis.

- [ ] **A**   Balanitis
- [ ] **B**   Hypospadias
- [ ] **C**   Non-retractile foreskin
- [ ] **D**   Paraphimosis
- [ ] **E**   Phimosis

CHAPTER 10 QUESTIONS

10.34 A 55-year-old man has uncontrolled hypertension. An ACE inhibitor (eg captopril) would be appropriate but he has moderate renal impairment.

Select the most appropriate advice from the list of options below.

- ☐ **A** Absolutely contraindicated
- ☐ **B** No change of dose required
- ☐ **C** Reduce dose
- ☐ **D** Reduce dose frequency
- ☐ **E** Relatively contraindicated

ANSWERS

THEME: LOW URINE OUTPUT AFTER SURGERY

10.1   E   Renal hypoperfusion due to hypotension

Epidural analgesia can reduce the blood pressure. This patient's usual dose of antihypertensive medication reduced the blood pressure even further, in this case leading to hypoperfusion of the kidneys which then produce less urine.

10.2   B   Acute urinary retention

Some older men will develop acute urinary retention following routine inguinal hernia surgery. This is thought to be due to a combination of prostatic hypertrophy and the anticholinergic effects of some anaesthetic reversal agents. Pain may also contribute. A brief period of catheterisation will usually be sufficient to treat the acute episode.

10.3   C   Blocked catheter

Clot retention is a common problem following TURP and often responds to bladder washout under strict aseptic technique. Rarely patients may need to return to theatre for further haemostatic diathermy.

10.4   A   Acute interstitial nephritis

Aminoglycoside antibiotics such as gentamicin can be nephrotoxic, as can non-steroidal anti-inflammatory drugs such as diclofenac. They can lead to acute renal failure due to interstitial nephritis. Risk factors for these effects include dehydration, hypotension, pre-existing renal impairment and the concomitant use of multiple nephrotoxic drugs.

THEME: INVESTIGATIONS FOR RENAL DISEASES

10.5 G Renal arteriography

When starting to take ACE inhibitors, patients should be advised that they will need to have blood tests for urea and creatinine at baseline, which will need to be repeated a week or two after starting the drug or following any dose increase. This is to monitor for the rare condition of renal artery stenosis, which can be revealed by ACE inhibitors (or angiotensin II receptor blockers). Patients with deteriorating urea and electrolyte findings should be investigated with renal arteriography to detect underlying arterial stenosis, as this can lead to chronic kidney disease if left undetected.

10.6 D Micturating cystography

The patient is screened during voiding after a contrast agent has been instilled into the bladder. This is to check for vesicoureteric reflux and to study urethral and bladder emptying.

10.7 B CT scan

CT can be used to detect lucent calculi. It is also used as first line to characterise renal masses that are indeterminate on ultrasound screening, for staging of renal tumours, evaluation of the retroperitoneum for tumours or fibrosis (that may be causing renal obstruction), assessment of renal trauma, and visualisation of renal vasculature.

10.8 K Ultrasound scan

Ultrasound is also useful for checking whether renal masses are solid or cystic, detecting infrarenal or perinephric fluid, and for demonstrating renal perfusion.

THEME: DIAGNOSIS OF RENAL DISEASE

10.9   I   Streptococcal glomerulonephritis

The incidence of streptococcal glomerulonephritis is declining in the West, but it is still prevalent in some parts of the world, particularly in tropical countries. It is due to the deposition of immune complexes in the glomeruli following infection with certain serotypes of *Streptococcus* that are mainly seen in those areas. It is not known why some people infected with the same serotypes do not have any sequelae. The condition typically affects children between 2 and 12 years.

10.10   C   Contrast medium-induced nephropathy

Some people are sensitive to the agents used as radiographic contrast. If someone has had recent investigations it is worth checking if they were given any injections during the procedure. Reactions can worsen on subsequent exposure, so patients should be clearly told to let radiographers know about this if they should need investigations in the future.

10.11   D   Haemolytic uraemic syndrome

Certain pathogens, including *Escherichia coli* serotype O157: H7, can produce 'verotoxins' that damage endothelial cells. This leads to platelet and fibrin deposition in small vessels, causing intravascular haemolysis. This is also known as microangiopathic haemolytic anaemia. The platelets are used up in the process (consumptive thrombocytopenia), and red cell degradation products damage the kidneys. It is a disease primarily of infancy and early childhood, and is the most common cause of acute renal failure in children.

10.12   H   Retroperitoneal fibrosis

This condition may extend from the level of the second lumbar vertebra to the pelvic brim. It is thought to be due to an autoimmune phenomenon. There is an association sometimes with abdominal aortic aneurysm but most cases are idiopathic. The differential diagnosis is retroperitoneal lymphoma.

THEME: MANAGEMENT OF ACUTE RENAL FAILURE

10.13   F   Haemofiltration

This patient can no longer be managed conservatively and needs to have more invasive treatment. His previous surgery makes CAPD unsuitable for him, therefore haemodialysis is the modality of choice.

10.14   C   Catheterisation

The patient's symptoms and biochemistry results are consistent with acute urinary retention causing obstructive uropathy. This may have been precipitated by treatment with diuretics for his heart failure, or a urinary tract infection. A brief period of catheterisation and careful fluid balance will usually help the renal function slowly return to his normal status.

10.15   I   Intravenous fluid

A large volume of fluid loss without adequate replacement can result in 'prenal' acute renal failure. This can be corrected by judicious fluid replacement.

10.16   B   Calcium resonium orally/per rectum

An ion-exchange resin such as calcium resonium can lower the potassium if the medications causing high levels cannot be stopped. If the patient had symptoms or there were electrocardiographic effects of hyperkalaemia he would need admission for intravenous treatment. However, with adequate monitoring, the oral or rectal route is acceptable in this situation.

THEME: MANAGEMENT OF CHRONIC KIDNEY DISEASE

10.17   C   Calcium/cholecalciferol supplements

At first diagnosis of stage 3 CKD, the PTH should be checked, and if it is raised the 25-hydroxyvitamin D should be checked. If this is low the patient should be started on ergo- or cholecalciferol plus calcium supplements (not calcium phosphate) in an attempt to maintain serum calcium concentrations in the normal range and prevent excess parathormone secretion.

10.18   D   Erythropoiesis-stimulating agents

The renal production of erythropoietin is reduced in CKD, therefore patients should be monitored for anaemia. In the absence of any other cause they should be treated with erythropoiesis-stimulating agents (eg epoetin or darbepoetin-α) to maintain the haemoglobin between 11.0g/l and 12.0g/l, depending on functional needs. These agents have side-effects including causing hypertension, and patients need to be monitored for this and treated accordingly.

10.19   H   Pneumococcal vaccine

Once a patient is diagnosed with CKD stage 3 or above, medications and vaccinations should be reviewed. Nephrotoxic drugs including non-steroidal anti-inflammatory drugs should be avoided if possible, and if the patient has never been given a pneumococcal vaccine this should be given as a single dose. The patient should also receive annual influenza vaccination.

10.20   G   Oral phosphodiesterase inhibitor

Phosphodiesterase inhibitors such as sildenafil can be effective in treating erectile dysfunction in patients with renal failure. These drugs are contraindicated in those receiving treatment with nitrates for coronary artery disease.

THEME: INCONTINENCE

10.21   G   Midstream sample of urine

Frequency and dysuria are classic symptoms of urinary tract infection. Occasionally the infection can cause detrusor irritability leading to urge incontinence. Treatment involves eradicating the infection. Unless the patient tells you she frequently suffers from cystitis it is appropriate to send a midstream sample of urine for culture and sensitivities prior to commencing empirical treatment.

10.22   I   Pelvic floor exercises

Following vaginal delivery, particularly if instrumental, there is damage to the pelvic floor muscles, which become overstretched and lax. It is important to advise the woman how to perform pelvic floor exercises, including giving information sheets with instructions.

10.23   B   Bladder training

Faecal overloading due to constipation can cause bladder outflow obstruction, leading to incomplete bladder emptying, frequency of micturition and sometimes overflow incontinence. Even though the obstruction has now cleared the bladder may take some time to get used to holding urine for longer periods once more. Bladder training, to extend the time between voids, can help this problem.

10.24   D   Colposuspension operation

In this situation it is appropriate to try pelvic floor exercises first, and then medication if this is unsuccessful.[1] A colposuspension procedure can provide support to the bladder neck and treat stress incontinence once other options have been exhausted.

THEME: PENILE AND SCROTAL LUMPS

10.25   B   Epididymal cyst

Epididymal cysts are common and often multiple. They usually present in middle age with a lump as in this case. Management involves reassuring the patient, an ultrasound may be needed if the diagnosis is uncertain. A spermatocele is similar to an epididymal cyst except that there is a connection to the testicle and the swelling is filled with cloudy fluid containing many sperm and sperm like cells.

10.26 I Testicular cancer

Because testicular cancer is curable when detected early, regular monthly testicular self-examination is recommend. Symptoms may include a lump or a hardening in one testis with abnormal sensitivity (numbness or pain) and/or a dull ache in the lower abdomen or groin. Occasionally there may be a generalised increase in size of the testicle or sometimes even a decrease in size. There may be loss of sexual activity, blood in the semen or hydrocele. The nature of any palpated lump in the scrotum is evaluated by scrotal ultrasound. The extent of the disease is evaluated by CT scans, which also locate metastases. Blood tests are used to identify and measure tumor markers that are specific to testicular cancer, AFP α-1 fetoprotein, β-HCG, and LDH. The diagnosis is made by performing an orchidectomy, along with attached structures.

10.27 J Testicular torsion

In testicular torsion the spermatic cord that carries the blood supply to a testicle is twisted, cutting off the blood supply leading, if prolonged, to the death of the testicle. The onset of pain is sudden and severe and there may also be pain in the corresponding iliac fossa. The patient may vomit. A Doppler ultrasound scan of the scrotum will show the presence or absence of blood flow to the testicle. With prompt diagnosis and treatment the testicle can be saved in a high number of cases. The scrotum is explored surgically, the testicle untwisted and protected from further torsion by attaching it to the scrotum wall. While torsion is more frequent among adolescents, it should be considered in all cases where there is testicular pain particularly when evidence of inflammation or infection is absent. Two risk factors are trauma and strenuous physical activity.

10.28 D Haematoma

Bruising and bleeding that may lead to the formation of a haematoma are common complications of vasectomy and patients should be warned.

10.29 H Sperm granuloma

There is an increase in pressure within the vas on the testicular side following vasectomy. The epididymides are often swollen and distended from back pressure. The efferent ducts and seminiferous tubules of the testes are also affected by back pressure, causing an increase in area and thickness. The thick muscle layers of the vas can easily become separated, leading to sperm buildup and extravasation. Cysts often form from the fluid that spreads between the layers. Sperm leaking from the vas and epididymides can form lesions in the scrotum known as sperm granulomas. Some sperm granulomas can be painful. This pain is often heightened during intercourse and ejaculation because, during ejaculation, muscles elevate the testis. The vas has two forms of electrical activity: pacesetter potentials and action potentials. After vasectomy, while the action potentials are diminished, the pacesetter potentials on the testicular side exhibit an irregular rhythm. This contributes to the pain syndrome. Also, nerves can become trapped in the fibrous tissue caused by vasectomy.

CHAPTER 10 ANSWERS

10.30 B Examine the patient, and do urinalysis

In April 2006 most laboratories started to routinely provide eGFR results with results of urea and electrolyte tests. It forms the basis of our diagnosis of chronic kidney disease (see the National Service Framework for referral criteria). The normal eGFR for a healthy young adult is above 90ml/min/1.73m^2. However, glomerular filtration rate slows with age, therefore a stable level between 60ml/min/1.73m^2 and 90ml/min/1.73m^2, with no other signs of kidney disease, may be acceptable and needs no further monitoring. It is calculated from the patient's creatinine. This means it is artificially lower in dehydration (such as during a fasting blood test; therefore advise patients to drink plenty of water).

For this patient it is important to exclude signs of chronic kidney disease such as proteinuria, oedema, enlarged kidneys on palpation, and potential causes of kidney damage such as severe hypertension or outflow obstruction from an enlarged prostate. In the absence of other signs or symptoms it would be appropriate to recheck the blood test in a month to ensure it is stable. This result may indicate his usual level of renal function secondary to long-term hypertension. ACE inhibitors would therefore be appropriate for him to prevent further damage, but should only be started once his baseline renal function is established, as this need to be monitored for any treatment-related deterioration.[2]

10.31   B   Finasteride plus tamsulosin

A number of predictive risk factors for both symptom progression and acute urinary retention (AUR) have been identified.[3] In this man both hesitancy and the moderate I-PSS score are risk factors for AUR as is a prostate volume exceeding 30cc, which presumably he has. I-PSS is a symptom index for benign prostatic hyperplasia that was developed and validated by a multidisciplinary measurement committee of the American Urological Association.[4] Scores range from 0–35 depending on symptoms and a score > 7 is associated with an increased risk of AUR.

Men with lower urinary symptoms and small or moderate prostates require only watchful waiting or if necessary α-blockers (eg tamsulosin) for symptom control. 5 α-reductase inhibitors (eg finasteride) reduce the risk of AUR and prostatectomy and therefore are indicated if risk factors are present. A combination with an α-blocker may be more beneficial than monotherapy. Surgical measures are indicated if medical treatment fails or cannot be tolerated or if there is another strong indicator such as refractory retention, bladder stones, renal insufficiency, recurrent UTIs or recurrent haematuria.

10.32   A   Fordyce's spots

They are common in men and women (on the labia) of all ages. The spots are a form of ectopic sebaceous gland, and are not known to be associated with any disease or illness and are of cosmetic concern only.

10.33   C   Non-retractile foreskin

It is normal for a baby's foreskin not to retract, but as the child grows the foreskin is expected to become retractable. Some have suggested that physiological infantile phimosis be referred to as developmental non-retractility of the foreskin to more clearly distinguish this from pathological form, which is known as phimosis. There is no deadline by which the foreskin should be retractable and often it does not occur until well into the teenage years. A non-retractable foreskin in a pre-pubescent child is not a disease and requires no treatment.

Paraphimosis is where the foreskin is retracted and becomes oedematous, making it unable to be replaced. It is an emergency and if gentle attempts to replace the foreskin with ice packs (to reduce swelling) and lubricant jelly are unsuccessful the child will require urgent referral. Balanitis is inflammation of the glans penis. Hypospadias is a birth defect of the urethra in the male that involves an abnormally placed urinary meatus.

10.34   C   Reduce dose

Captopril may become toxic if creatinine clearance is low. The risk of cardiovascular side-effects is greater. The starting dose should be reduced and the patient's renal function should be monitored more regularly. Angiotensin-converting enzyme (ACE) inhibitors are contraindicated in patients with bilateral renal artery stenosis or unilateral renal artery stenosis supplying a single functioning kidney. In these situations, reduction in angiotensin II may lead to rapid deterioration in renal function. Particular care should be taken in prescribing NSAIDS in combination with ACE inhibitors. Creatinine clearance in patients with renal artery stenosis may be well preserved and serum creatinine may be normal. ACE inhibitors are being used increasingly by renal specialists for controlling hypertension in patients with renal disease with good evidence of a protective effect.

CHAPTER 10 ANSWERS

REFERENCES

1. National Institute for Health and Clinical Excellence. *Urinary incontinence: the management of urinary incontinence in women* (homepage on the Internet), Octoberr 2006 (cited 2008 May 2). Available from http://www.nice.org.uk/cg40

2. Department of Health. *National Service Framework for Renal Services: Part 2 – chronic kidney disease, acute renal failure and end of life care.* February 2005.

3. British Assocation of Urological Surgeons. *Primary care management of male lower urinary tract symptoms (LUTS).* February 2004.

4. The American Urological Association symptom index for benign prostatic hyperplasia. The Measurement Committee of the American Urological Association. J Urol 1992 Nov;148(5): 1549–57.

Chapter 11
Reproductive

QUESTIONS

THEME: GYNAECOLOGICAL INVESTIGATIONS

Options

A Cervical punch biopsy

B Colposcopy and large loop excision of the transformation zone

C Diagnostic hysteroscopy and endometrial biopsy

D Diagnostic laparoscopy and tubal dye test

E Diagnostic laparotomy

F Hysterosalpingo contrast sonography (HyCoSy)

G Hysterosalpingography

H Pregnancy test and serum β-human chorionic gonadotrophin

I Serum luteinising hormone (LH) and serum follicle-stimulating hormone (FSH)

J Transabdominal ultrasound of the pelvis

K Transvaginal ultrasound of the pelvis, Pipelle biopsy and saline sonography

For each of the patients below, choose the single most appropriate investigation from the list of options above. Each option may be used once, more than once or not at all.

☐ **11.1** **A 55-year-old woman presents with intermenstrual bleeding while on cyclical combined hormone replacement therapy.**

☐ **11.2** A 23-year-old woman is rushed into the Emergency Department in a state of shock. Her partner informs you that she had been complaining of lower abdominal pain this morning and then suddenly collapsed. He also tells you that her last menstrual period was 6–7 weeks ago. A portable transabdominal scan (TAS) shows free fluid in the pelvis. On examination her Glasgow Coma Score is 3, pulse is 140bpm, blood pressure is 70/40mmHg.

☐ **11.3** A 35-year-old woman presents with a 2-year history of primary subfertility. She also gives a history of menstrual irregularity, severe dysmenorrhoea and dyspareunia.

☐ **11.4** A 42-year-old woman presents with a 4-year history of secondary infertility. She already has a 6-year-old girl who was conceived through in vitro fertilisation. It has only been recently that she has had the financial means to consider a second child. She also informs you that for the past few months her periods have gradually become more and more irregular and she has also been experiencing night sweats.

☐ **11.5** A 48-year-old asylum seeker presents with a history of bloodstained, foul-smelling vaginal discharge. On per speculum examination you see a large ulcerated mass arising from the cervix.

CHAPTER 11 QUESTIONS

THEME: CONTRACEPTION

Options

A Combined oral contraceptive
B Condoms
C Dianette
D Diaphragm with spermicidal gel
E Implanon
F Injection of Depo-Provera
G Intrauterine copper device
H Lactational amenorrhoea method (LAM)
I Levonorgestrel (morning-after pill)
J Mirena coil
K Progesterone-only pill

For each of the patients below, choose the single most appropriate method of contraception from the list of options above. Each option may be used once, more than once or not at all.

☐ **11.6** An 18-year-old girl comes to your family planning clinic requesting contraceptive advice. She has been sexually active for the past year and is in a stable relationship with her boyfriend. She also informs you that she does not want anything that will make her acne worse. It has failed to respond to a 6-month course of erythromycin.

☐ **11.7** A 26-year-old woman, 7 weeks' postpartum, comes to your family planning clinic for contraceptive advice. While taking a history you gather she is fully breastfeeding. She is not keen on any hormonal contraceptive, as her best friends have told her that they can reduce breast milk.

☐ **11.8** A 24-year-old woman tourist is brought into the Emergency Department by the police surgeon who provides information that she was raped 4 days ago. You are asked to perform a medical examination on the patient and advise her about the most suitable contraception. Her last menstrual period was 12 days ago and she has a regular 28-day cycle.

☐ **11.9** A 45-year-old woman is requesting sterilisation. Her history reveals that she has been happily married for the past 20 years and her husband is not keen on a vasectomy. She also tells you that she has recently noticed that her periods have become heavier and puts this down to her increased weight. Her present body mass index is 38.

☐ **11.10** A 35-year-old woman has five children and does not want any more. Her last two pregnancies were conceived after contraception failure, while on the pill and the injection. Her records reveal she had tested positive for *Chlamydia* and was seen in the genitourinary medicine clinic 2 years ago.

THEME: VAGINAL BLEEDING IN PREGNANCY

Options

A Abortion (complete)

B Abortion (incomplete)

C Abortion (missed)

D Abortion (threatened)

E Cervicitis

F Ectopic pregnancy

G Hydatidiform mole

H Labour

I Placenta praevia

J Placental abruption

K Uterine rupture

For each of the patients below, choose the single most likely diagnosis from the list of options above. Each option may be used once, more than once or not at all.

☐ **11.11** A woman 35 weeks' pregnant rapidly develops severe constant lower abdominal pain and vaginal blood loss. The uterus is hard and tender, BP 80/55, pulse 125/min and temperature 37°C. The fetal heart is not heard.

☐ **11.12** A woman 10 weeks' pregnant has small amounts of intermittent blood loss over 2 days without pain. The cervical os is not dilated and uterine size approximately 10 weeks.

☐ **11.13** A woman 14 weeks' pregnant has painless vaginal bleeding. She has been vomiting throughout the pregnancy. The fundus is 18 weeks in size and her blood pressure is 140/90. A blood test shows high levels of human chorionic gonadotrophin.

☐ **11.14** A woman 37 weeks' pregnant has had regular pains and uterine tightening every 15 minutes over 3 hours with blood stained mucus discharge. Abdominal and obstetric examination is normal. The fetal head is engaged.

☐ **11.15** A woman 12 weeks' pregnant reports the passage of 'tissue' and blood from the vagina accompanied by lower abdominal pain. She continues to bleed. The cervical os is open.

THEME: VAGINAL DISCHARGE

Options

A   Atrophic vaginitis

B   Bacterial vaginosis

C   Candidiasis

D   Cervical cancer

E   Ectropion

F   Foreign body

G   Gonorrhoea

H   Mittelschmerz

I   Non-gonococcal urethritis (NGU)

J   Non-specific vulvovaginitis

K   *Trichomonas vaginalis* infection

For each of the patients below, choose the single most appropriate diagnosis from the list of options above. Each option may be used once, more than once or not at all.

☐ **11.16**   A 5-year-old girl is brought by her mother to the walk-in clinic. The mother informs you that she has been recently noticing a discharge on the girl's undergarments. On examination of the external genitalia you notice it to be red and inflamed.

☐ **11.17**   A 65-year-old woman comes to have her ring pessary changed. Her history reveals that, although she has been well with regard to her prolapse, she has recently been having some bloodstained discharge.

☐ **11.18** A 23-year-old woman attends the GP surgery complaining of an itchy vaginal discharge. She is in a stable relationship and does not take any contraceptive pill. On examination you notice red and oedematous labia with white spongy areas.

☐ **11.19** An 18-year-old woman comes to the GP surgery complaining of excessive clear vaginal discharge. She is on the combined pill and describes her symptoms as 'feeling wet all the time'.

☐ **11.20** A 26-year-old woman comes to the clinic complaining of dysuria and painful intercourse. She also says she has been recently getting a funny vaginal discharge. She described it as being frothy with a musty smell, causing intense itching and soreness in her vagina.

THEME: VULVAL DISORDERS

Options

A   Behçet's disease
B   Candidiasis
C   Carcinoma of the vulva
D   Condyloma lata
E   Herpes simplex
F   Lichen sclerosus
G   Sebaceous cyst
H   Tinea cruris
I   Varicose veins
J   Vulval abscess
K   Vulval psoriasis
L   Vulval wart

For each of the patients below, choose the single most appropriate diagnosis from the list of options above. Each option may be used once, more than once or not at all.

☐ **11.21** A 55-year-old woman complains of vaginal bleeding. She has recently noticed a small ulcer on her genitals. On examination there is an ulcer on the vulva, which has an indurated base and everted margins. Palpation reveals inguinal lymphadenopathy.

☐ **11.22** A 30-year-old 7 month's pregnant woman comes to the antenatal clinic complaining of a bluish lump that she has noticed in her vulva. The lump has gradually increased in size but has remained painless.

☐ **11.23** A 28-year-old woman has noticed white patches, which are itchy, on her vulva. On examination you notice white atrophic areas on the vulval skin.

☐ **11.24** A 20-year-old patient, 6 months' pregnant, attends the genitourinary medicine clinic having been referred by the community midwife after noticing warty lesions on her vulva. On taking a history you gather she is in a stable relationship and has noticed this growth only in the past few weeks. She has no history of having a sexually transmitted infection in the past.

☐ **11.25** A 32-year-old woman is referred by her GP with a painful vulval swelling, which has become progressively larger and has now burst. On examining her you notice a lump in the labia majora. The lump has a punctum and is discharging foul-smelling pus.

☐ **11.26** A 40-year old woman has well demarcated non-scaly erythema involving the vulva and extending to the intertriginous skin of the groin. She also has thick scaling on the scalp.

THEME: TREATMENT WITH HORMONES

Options

A   Combined oral contraceptive

B   Continuous combined oestrogen/progesterone

C   Oestrogen (tablets or patch)

D   Progesterone (depot injection)

E   Progesterone (tablets)

F   Sequential combined oestrogen/progesterone

G   Vaginal oestrogen

H   None of these

For each patient below select the single most suitable treatment from the list above. Each option may be used once, more than once or not at all.

☐ **11.27** A 17-year-old woman is going on holiday for one week. Her period is due to start on the first day of her holiday and she wishes to postpone menstruation. She does not take an oral contraceptive.

☐ **11.28** A 48-year-old woman is bothered by hot flushes. They are embarrassing at meetings and also affect her sleep. She still has a period most months.

☐ **11.29** A 54-year-old woman has frequent hot flushes. Her periods stopped 3 years ago.

☐ **11.30** A 58-year-old woman has an osteoporotic crush fracture of a dorsal vertebra. She had a hysterectomy at the age of 45 years.

☐ **11.31** A 19-year-old woman is troubled with dysmenorrhoea. She has tried mefenamic acid and claims it was 'useless'. You have had doubts in the past about her compliance with treatment.

11.32 A 26-year-old woman, 28 weeks' pregnant, complains of breathlessness during a routine antenatal check-up. On clinical examination everything is normal except she is slightly hyperventilating.

Which one of the following findings would you be surprised to encounter during a normal pregnancy?

- ☐ **A** Decrease in the serum ferritin level
- ☐ **B** Increase in cardiac output
- ☐ **C** Increase in glomerular filtration rate (GFR)
- ☐ **D** Increase in the levels of clotting factors VII, VIII and IX
- ☐ **E** Increase in total lung capacity

11.33 A 26-year-old woman and her 28-year-old partner come to see the GP surgery complaining of primary infertility for 2 years. She gives a history of irregular menstrual cycles.

What one of the following is the single best test to see whether she is ovulating or not?

- ☐ **A** Basal body temperature estimation
- ☐ **B** Cervical fern test
- ☐ **C** Day-2 LH and FSH
- ☐ **D** Day-21 progesterone level
- ☐ **E** Endometrial biopsy

11.34 A 32-year-old pregnant woman presented to her GP with pruritus during the third trimester. Liver biochemistry shows cholestasis.

Which one of the following is the single most likely outcome?

☐ **A** The condition will not resolve after delivery

☐ **B** The fetus will probably be harmed

☐ **C** The ingestion of oestrogen-containing oral contraceptive pills will decrease the risk

☐ **D** The prognosis for the mother is poor

☐ **E** There is a minimal risk of recurrence in subsequent pregnancies

11.35 A 32-year-old woman has a 4-month history of amenorrhoea after stopping the combined oral contraceptive. She is recently married and very concerned as she wants to conceive.

Which one of the following is the most appropriate next course of action?

☐ **A** Follicle-stimulating hormone (FSH) and luteinising hormone (LH) level measurements

☐ **B** Pelvic ultrasound

☐ **C** Pregnancy test

☐ **D** Review in 2 months without further tests

☐ **E** Thyroid function tests

11.36 Identify from the list below the single intervention that is felt to be of value as a component of routine antenatal care.

☐ **A** Iron supplements

☐ **B** Pelvic examination

☐ **C** Regular dipstick testing for glycosuria

☐ **D** Regular maternal weighing

☐ **E** Screening for asymptomatic bacteriuria

ANSWERS

THEME: GYNAECOLOGICAL INVESTIGATIONS

11.1 **K** **Transvaginal ultrasound of the pelvis, Pipelle biopsy and saline sonography**

Although one might think that any of options C, J, or K may be right, in the NHS setting this is the most appropriate answer. Most hospitals have these one-stop 'postmenopausal bleeding clinics' where the diagnostic procedures are performed on an outpatient basis. Sonohysterography is gradually replacing outpatient hysteroscopy as it can be combined with the scan to give a more detailed pelvic assessment. It is also more patient friendly. The most likely diagnosis in this case is endometrial polyp, which is common in women using combined hormone replacement therapy.

11.2 **E** **Diagnostic laparotomy**

This is a scenario of ruptured ectopic pregnancy and E is the only possible answer. It is the only life-threatening gynaecological emergency that requires immediate surgery.

11.3 **D** **Diagnostic laparoscopy and tubal dye test**

The symptoms described here by the patient point towards endometriosis. Although both transvaginal HyCoSy and HSG (hysterosalpingogram) help in diagnosing tubal and other uterine structural problems, they cannot assess the pelvis to diagnose endometriosis. Hence, it may be worthwhile to first think of the disease and then work out the best diagnostic modality in the given scenario.

11.4   I   Serum LH and serum FSH

This is because there is suspicion of premature ovarian failure based on the symptoms.

11.5   A   Cervical punch biopsy

This is obviously a case of suspected cervical malignancy that needs to be ruled out by tissue biopsy. As the patient is an asylum seeker it means she is not in the National Cervical Screening Programme.

THEME: CONTRACEPTION

11.6   C   Dianette

Dianette is the trade name for co-cyprindiol, which is a mixture of cyproterone acetate 2mg and ethinylestradiol 35µg. This is an antiandrogen and reduces acne by decreasing the sebum secretion, which is under androgen control. Dianette is the only licensed drug for acne and hirsutism in the UK. It is ideal for people who need contraception and for whom acne is also a problem. Venous thromboembolism occurs more frequently in those taking Dianette than those taking a low-dose combined oral contraceptive. The Committee on Safety of Medicines (CSM) advises that Dianette is licensed for severe acne that has not responded to oral antibiotics and should not be used solely for contraception. It is contraindicated where there is a personal or close family history of venous thromboembolism.[1]

11.7   H   Lactational amenorrhoea method (LAM)

The lactational amenorrhoea method (LAM) can be considered when the mother is fully breastfeeding. It is based on the physiologic effect of suckling to suppress ovulation. Women may be advised that if they are less than 6 months' postpartum, amenorrhoeic and fully breastfeeding (at the very least, breastfeed for almost all feedings), the LAM is over 98% effective in preventing pregnancy. The progestogen-only contraceptive is an alternative. This does not affect the volume of breast milk and provides 99% contraceptive efficacy when breastfeeding.

11.8   G   Intrauterine copper device

A copper intrauterine contraceptive device (IUCD) can be inserted up to 5 days following unprotected intercourse at any time in the menstrual cycle provided this is the only unprotected sex that has occurred since the last period. If there has been unprotected sex more than once since the last period then the IUCD can be fitted up to 5 days after the earliest time ovulation could have occurred (day 14 in a 28-day cycle).

The 'morning-after pill' is also known as 'post-coital contraception' and the recommended method is one dose of Levonelle (levonorgestrel 1500μg) taken as soon as possible after unprotected intercourse. If taken within 24 hours it will prevent up to 95% of pregnancies, and up to 85% if taken between 24 and 48 hours. If taken between 49 and 72 hours it will prevent up to 58% of pregnancies. It is only licensed to be taken within 72 hours of unprotected intercourse, as the efficacy after this is unknown.

11.9   J   Mirena coil

Considering the patient's age, her high BMI and menstrual problems this seems the best option. The Mirena coil is a progesterone-only intrauterine system that releases 20μg of levonorgestrel directly into the uterine cavity every 24 hours. It acts by preventing endometrial proliferation and is very effective in controlling menorrhagia.

CHAPTER 11 ANSWERS

11.10   E   Implanon

This patient has a problem with contraceptive compliance and needs reliable long-term contraception. Taking into consideration that she has had a sexually transmitted infection in the past, IUCD would not be ideal for her. Although you can consider condoms, her history of poor compliance with the pill and injections and also the poor efficacy of condoms will not make these an ideal choice for her. Implanon is an implant containing a progesterone contraceptive. It contains etonogestrel, is subdermally implanted and is effective for 3 years. It also has a very low Pearl Index (ie the measure of contraceptive efficacy expressed in 100 women-reproductive years). She should be advised that nuisance bleeding can occur, particularly in the first few months after insertion.

THEME: VAGINAL BLEEDING IN PREGNANCY

11.11   J   Placental abruption

This condition occurs when a placenta separates from the wall of the uterus after 20 weeks of gestation and blood collects between the placenta and the uterus. Such separation occurs in 1 in 200 of all pregnancies. The cause is unknown. Risk factors for placental abruption include high blood pressure (140/90 or greater), trauma, cocaine or tobacco use and abruption in previous pregnancy. It occurs in 1% of pregnancies world-wide with a fetal mortality rate of 20–40% depending on the degree of separation. Placental abruption can also cause maternal death. Placental abruption is suspected when a pregnant woman has sudden localised uterine pain with or without bleeding. The fundal height may be monitored because a rising fundus can be a sign of bleeding.

11.12   D   Abortion (threatened)

Vaginal bleeding occurs in 25% of first trimester pregnancies with up to half of these progressing to miscarriage. It follows that many do not abort. A healthy pregnancy can be confirmed by transvaginal ultrasound.

11.13 G Hydatidiform mole

Molar pregnancy is an abnormal pregnancy, characterised by the presence of an abnormal growth containing a non-viable embryo, which implants and grows within the uterus. There is an increased trophoblast proliferation and enlargening of chorionic villi. Angiogenesis in the trophoblasts is impaired as well. The mole is removed upon diagnosis because there is risk of developing into choriocarcinoma. The diagnosis is strongly suggested by ultrasound but definitive diagnosis requires histopathological examination. The mole resembles a bunch of grapes. Sometimes symptoms of hyperthyroidism are seen, due to very high levels of HCG, which can behave like thyroid-stimulating hormone (TSH).

11.14 H Labour

One of the first signs that labour may soon be starting is a 'show'. This is a blood-streaked mucus plug which is passed out of the vagina when the cervix begins to change. This is not a very reliable sign and not all women see this. For those women who do see a show, labour may be as much as two weeks away.

The most common indication that labour has begun is the start of painful contractions. These can range in intensity from mild irritation to strong pain and may be felt low down in the back or like waves moving across the abdomen. When contractions are regular (coming every 5–10 minutes), and lasting 45–60 seconds then labour is established. The contractions of labour are not to be confused with Braxton Hicks contractions. These intermittent contractions of the uterus occur all through pregnancy, but become more obvious as pregnancy progresses. They are usually painless.

Another sign of labour is rupture of the membranes. This can happen before labour starts, before painful contractions. Sometimes this can be confused with a loss of urine.

11.15 B Abortion (incomplete)

When pieces of tissue are too large for the uterus to expel it creates a situation where the uterus is not able to contract to its normal size with the result that haemorrhage continues. It can be heavy or it may cause prolonged bleeding lasting 2 or more weeks with bleeding moderate or light. Incomplete abortion can also manifest in ways other than haemorrhage. It can become infected leading to fever or more widespread pelvic inflammatory disease. Early evacuation of retained products of conception is the treatment of choice.

THEME: VAGINAL DISCHARGE

11.16 J Non-specific vulvovaginitis

This is the commonest gynaecological problem in the prepubertal age group. Due to low levels of oestrogen between birth and puberty, the vaginal mucosa is thin and alkaline, making it less resistant to bacteria. Management takes the form of reassuring anxious parents, maintaining good hygiene and wearing loose-fitting cotton undergarments. If infection is present Group A β-haemolytic streptococcus is not an uncommon cause. Candida vulvovaginitis is extremely uncommon in the prepubertal child who is no longer wearing nappies. It must be remembered however that some children do wear nappies at night only (nocturnal enuresis) until they are well beyond 5 years of age and they may be susceptible to a candida vulvovaginitis. Other organisms are unusual and must raise the possibility of sexual abuse.

11.17 A Atrophic vaginitis

It is due to post-menopausal oestrogen lack. This is a classic presentation. The dry, thin, atrophic vaginal mucosa rubs against the undergarments and causes bleeding and staining.

11.18   C   Candidiasis

This is a typical picture of vulval candidiasis and can be treated with clotrimazole pessaries or vaginal cream, or with a single dose of fluconazole 150mg orally. It is also important to treat the partner to prevent reinfection.

11.19   E   Ectropion

This is the commonest cause of a clear, non-itchy vaginal discharge. This is common among pill users as it induces the columnar epithelium to spread over the transformation zone of the cervix. Columnar epithelium is secretory.

11.20   K   *Trichomonas vaginalis* infection

This is a typical discharge found in these infections. On per speculum examination the cervix is seen to have multiple small haemorrhagic areas, which lead to the description 'strawberry cervix'. Metronidazole 400mg, twice/thrice a day for 7 days is the treatment of choice. It is important to take swabs to check sensitivities, and to screen for other sexually transmitted infections. Partner notification is also important.

THEME: VULVAL DISORDERS

11.21   C   Carcinoma of the vulva

The presence of such a characteristic ulcer with lymphadenopathy is diagnostic of a cancerous lesion.

11.22   J   Varicose veins

Vulval varicosity is worsened in pregnancy due to the pressure of the gravid uterus obstructing venous drainage from the lower extremity.

CHAPTER 11 ANSWERS

11.23   F   Lichen sclerosus

The older terms that might have been used to describe these lesions, such as vulvar dystrophy, kraurosis vulvae, leukoplakia, hyperplastic vulvitis, and lichen sclerosus et atrophicus, should no longer be used. They are now non-neoplastic epithelial disorders, which are divided into three major categories: squamous cell hyperplasia, lichen sclerosus, and other dermatoses. The only sure way to differentiate is by histology. If atypical cells are present, the diagnosis is vulvar intraepithelial neoplasia. A further classification puts lichen sclerosus under inflammatory skin conditions, further grouped as a lichenoid disorder, while squamous hyperplasia is under psoriasiform disorders as lichenification, encompassing the term lichen simplex. Unfortunately, although the terminology may be comprehensive, it does not clarify the link with vulvar cancer. The latter seems to be an uncommon complication. For treatment, clobetasol propionate 0.05% ointment is applied twice daily. Because the effect is usually good, use is usually tapered off after 2–3 weeks. Indefinite maintenance continues with small amounts in many cases.

11.24   L   Vulval wart

Vulval warts are caused by the human papillomavirus (HPV). They become more florid in immunosuppressed conditions such as pregnancy. Certain serotypes have been implicated in cervical intraepithelial neoplasia and there is now a vaccine to prevent infection with these. The warts are sexually transmitted.

11.25   G   Sebaceous cyst

This is a typical presentation and the patient is often referred by the GP with a diagnosis of Bartholin abscess.

CHAPTER 11 ANSWERS

11.26   K   Vulval psoriasis

Psoriasis at this site is usually not scaly but still has the sharp demarcated edge of plaque psoriasis elsewhere. In candidiasis usually there are satellite lesions and in tinea cruris the margins are scaly and there is central clearing.

THEME: TREATMENT WITH HORMONES

11.27   E   Progesterone (tablets)

A suitable treatment would be norethisterone tablets 5mg three times a day starting 3 days before the expected start of the period and continuing until she wants to start the period, ie the end of the holiday. Had she been taking an oral contraceptive the simple solution would have been not to have had the normal pill break between packets of pills, ie start the next packet the day after finishing the current one.

11.28   F   Sequential combined oestrogen/progesterone

The majority of sequential combined HRT regimens are designed to mimic the menstrual cycle and so result in monthly bleeds. Oestrogen is taken continuously with progesterone added for the last 10–14 days. Generally packs are based on a 28-day cycle but long-cycle regimens are available for women who have only infrequent bleeds to give them a period every 3 months.

11.29   B   Continuous combined oestrogen/progesterone

Here oestrogen and progesterone are taken together daily with no break so that no bleeding will occur. However, there may be some initial breakthrough bleeding. Endometrial assessment should be considered if bleeding becomes heavier or continues after 6 months or resumes after a period of amenorrhoea.

11.30   H   None of these

Oestrogen reduces the rate of bone breakdown and so helps prevent osteoporosis. A woman without a uterus could take unopposed oestrogen. Progesterone is added only to protect against endometrial cancer, which is a potential problem with unopposed oestrogen. Protection against osteoporosis requires long-term HRT and bone breakdown recommences when HRT is stopped. The increased risk of developing breast cancer with HRT is related to the duration of use and for this reason the CSM has advised that HRT no longer be a first-line treatment for osteoporosis.[2]

11.31   D   Progesterone (depot injection)

Oral contraceptives can improve or relieve symptoms of primary dysmenorrhoea. The mechanism of action involves reducing menstrual blood volume, and suppressing ovulation. It may take up to 3 months of treatment to obtain relief. Doubts about her compliance make this a less attractive option than depot progesterone. This is effective since it usually induces amenorrhoea. The IntraUterine System (Mirena IUD) has been cited as useful in reducing symptoms of dysmenorrhoea in suitable patients.

11.32   E   Increase in total lung capacity

Total lung capacity is decreased in pregnancy by about 200ml. This is because the residual volume is reduced by 200ml, secondary to the large intra-abdominal swelling in pregnancy.

11.33   D   Day 21 progesterone level

This is the easiest test to check the ovulatory status. If the day 21 progesterone results are > 30nmol/l in two cycles, the woman is ovulating.

11.34   B   The fetus will probably be harmed

Intrahepatic cholestasis of pregnancy carries an increased risk of premature labour, fetal and maternal haemorrhaging, fetal distress, and intrauterine death of baby. Pruritus typically develops after 20 weeks of pregnancy, is prominent on the arms, legs and trunk, and progresses until delivery. Jaundice may develop 2–4 weeks later without progressing. The pathogenesis of intrahepatic cholestasis of pregnancy is unclear. Multiple factors probably interact with a genetic predisposition to alter the membrane composition of bile ducts and hepatocytes and increase their sensitivity to sex steroids. Close monitoring of fetal wellbeing is essential, although no single test reliably predicts the risk of intrauterine death and early delivery may be desirable. Recurrent cholestasis may occur during subsequent pregnancies or if patients take combined oral contraceptives.

11.35   C   Pregnancy test

If the patient has not done a pregnancy test then this needs to be done first. Secondary amenorrhoea is due to pregnancy until proved otherwise. Even denial of sexual activity should be taken with a degree of circumspection. 'Post-pill amenorrhoea' occurs when stopping oral contraceptives does not lead to a resumption of a normal menstrual cycle. It usually settles spontaneously in about 3 months but if not it will need to be investigated. The condition is probably not a true entity as the cause of amenorrhoea started while taking the contraceptives. These induced an artificial cycle until they were stopped.

11.36   E   Screening for asymptomatic bacteriuria

Asymptomatic bacteriuria occurs in 2–10% of pregnancies and, if not treated, up to 30% of mothers will develop acute pyelonephritis. Asymptomatic bacteriuria has been associated with low birthweight and preterm delivery. Screening for asymptomatic bacteriuria with urine culture and treatment with antibiotics is recommended during pregnancy, because it significantly reduces symptomatic urinary tract infections, low birth weight, and preterm delivery.[3] The presence of simultaneous pyuria does not warrant treatment by itself.

REFERENCES

1.   *Oral preparations for acne.* 13.6.2. British National Formulary; 55; 2008.

2.   Medicines and Healthcare products Regulatory Agency. *Hormone replacement therapy (HRT).* (homepage on the Internet), February 2008 (cited 2008 May 4). Available from http://www.mhra.gov.uk/Safetyinformation/Safetywarningsalertsandrecalls/Safetywarningsandmessagesformedicines/CON2015689

3.   Smaill F, Vazquez JC. Antibiotics for asymptomatic bacteriuria in pregnancy. Cochrane Database Syst Rev. 2007; (2):CD000490.

CHAPTER 11 ANSWERS

Chapter 12
Respiratory

QUESTIONS

THEME: SPIROMETRY

Options

A Bronchial challenge test
B FEV_1
C FEV_1/FVC
D FVC
E Reversibility test

The options above are terms used in spirometry. Select the single option that applies to each statement below. Each option may be used once, more than once or not at all.

☐ **12.1** Indicates an obstructive pattern if it is < 80% of the predicted value for age, sex and size

☐ **12.2** This is the total amount of air that can be blown out in one breath

☐ **12.3** Usually normal in a restrictive pattern of pulmonary disease

☐ **12.4** Can be used to distinguish asthma from chronic obstructive pulmonary disease (COPD)

THEME: MANAGEMENT OF CHRONIC OBSTRUCTIVE PULMONARY DISEASE

Options

A Amoxicillin

B Beclometasone inhaler

C Influenza vaccine

D Oxygen (long term)

E Pneumococcal vaccine

F Regular nebulised salbutamol

G Salmeterol

H Tiotropium

I Zarfilukast

The options above are drugs that may be used in the management of chronic obstructive pulmonary disease (COPD). Select the single option that applies to each statement below. Each option may be used once, more than once or not at all.

☐ **12.5** **Reduces exacerbations of COPD**

☐ **12.6** **Use only during exacerbations**

☐ **12.7** **Recommended when the FEV$_1$ is < 50% (severe COPD) and there are frequent exacerbations**

☐ **12.8** **Can be added to regular salmeterol in patients with moderate COPD**

☐ **12.9** **Indicated only in severe COPD and reduces mortality**

THEME: MANAGEMENT OF ADULT ASTHMA

Options

A Beclometasone 400µg/day
B Beclometasone 800µg/day
C Beclometasone 2000µg/day
D Ipratropium bromide 120µg/day
E Montelukast 10mg/day
F Prednisolone 5mg daily
G Prednisolone 40mg daily for 5 days
H Salbutamol 200µg as required
I Salmeterol 100µg daily

For each patient below, choose the single most suitable option from the above list. Each option may be used once, more than once or not at all.

☐ **12.10** A 35-year old woman's asthma has become less troublesome. She needs her bronchodilator infrequently. She uses beclometasone 800µg per day.

☐ **12.11** A 25-year-old man has frequent exercise-induced asthma and occasionally finds his asthma wakes him. His medication consists of salmeterol 100µg/day, beclometasone 400µg/day and he frequently needs to use his short-acting bronchodilator.

☐ **12.12** A 40-year-old woman's asthma is poorly controlled in spite of salmeterol 100µg/day, beclometasone 2000µg/day as well as a short-acting bronchodilator.

☐ **12.13** A 45-year-old woman is having frequent acute exacerbations of asthma. She uses salmeterol 100µg/day, beclometasone 2000µg/day as well as a short-acting bronchodilator and slow-release theophylline 500mg per day.

☐ **12.14** A 20-year-old woman wheezes when her hay fever is bad. It sometimes disturbs sleep.

☐ **12.15** A 50-year-old man is having an acute severe attack. He has an increased respiratory rate, a pulse of 112/minute and cannot finish a sentence in one breath.

THEME: DIAGNOSIS OF RESPIRATORY DISORDERS

Options

A	Bronchiectasis	E	Pleural effusion
B	Cystic fibrosis	F	Pulmonary embolism
C	Extrinsic allergic alveolitis	G	Sarcoidosis
D	Idiopathic pulmonary fibrosis	H	Spontaneous pneumothorax

For each of the patients below, choose the single most appropriate diagnosis from the list of options above. Each option may be used once, more than once or not at all.

☐ **12.16** A 25-year-old man experiences left sided chest pain and dyspnoea of sudden onset. There are diminished breath sounds over the whole of the left lung and percussion note is hyper-resonant.

☐ **12.17** A 62-year-old man has a cough, dyspnoea, right-sided chest pain, and weight loss. Symptoms have slowly worsened over 4 weeks. There are diminished breath sounds over the right lower lobe and the percussion note is dull.

☐ **12.18** A 35-year-old man presents with a flu-like illness with fever, chest tightness, dry cough and dyspnoea. There are inspiratory crepitations at both lung bases. This is the third time you have seen him with such an illness. He runs a livery stable for horses.

☐ **12.19** A 48-year-old woman has had frequent chest infections over the last 5 years. She coughs up large amounts of purulent sputum that is sometimes blood stained. An X-ray 6 months previously was reported to be normal. She has a faint wheeze.

☐ **12.20** A 22-year-old woman has tender indurated inflammatory nodules in the pretibial regions of both lower legs as well as arthralgia. Routine chest X-ray reveals bilateral hilar lymphadenopathy.

THEME: PNEUMONIA

Options

A Cytomegalovirus
B *Klebsiella pneumoniae*
C *Legionella pneumophila*
D *Mycoplasma pneumoniae*
E *Pneumocystis jiroveci*
F *Pseudomonas aeruginosa*
G Streptococcal pneumonia
H Tuberculosis

For each of the patients below, choose the single most appropriate answer from the list of options above. Each option may be used once, more than once or not at all.

CHAPTER 12 QUESTIONS

☐ **12.21** A 56-year-old man with no underlying lung problems went on holiday to Cyprus. He developed a dry cough and cold, which seemed like a viral prodromal illness. After 4–5 days he felt confused and started with diarrhoea and vomiting. A blood test shows a white blood cell count of 11.6 x 10^9/l, neutrophils 10.1 x 10^9/l, lymphocytes 0.7 x 10^9/l, eosinophils 0.3 x 10^9/l, monocytes 0.5 x 10^9/l. He is also found to have hyponatraemia, hypoalbuminaemia and a high level of aspartate aminotransferase (AST).

☐ **12.22** A 70-year-old woman with known chronic obstructive pulmonary disease and diabetes presents with increased shortness of breath, some streaky haemoptysis and a cough that produces purulent green sputum. She is also a known alcoholic. Her chest X-ray revealed extensive bilateral consolidation.

☐ **12.23** A 22-year-old man with known cystic fibrosis presents with a cough and breathlessness, which are much worse than usual.

☐ **12.24** A 16-year-old boy living in an institution presents with headache and malaise that preceded a dry cough by 48 hours. He has also developed a rash, predominantly on his arms and legs. Blood tests show his haemoglobin to be 10.1g/dl, with a reticulocyte count of 5% and thrombocytopenia. His chest X-ray shows bilateral extensive shadowing in both lungs.

☐ **12.25** A 58-year-old renal transplant recipient who is on ciclosporin has developed a high fever, severe breathlessness and a dry cough. His chest X-ray shows mild shadowing in the perihilar region on the right side. Pulse oximetry demonstrates gross desaturation on air.

THEME: BLOOD GAS ANALYSIS

Options

A Diabetes

B Head injury

C Mild asthma

D Paracetamol poisoning

E Primary hyperventilation

F Pulmonary embolism

G Severe asthma

H Tension pneumothorax

For each of the following blood gas results, select the single most likely diagnosis from the list of options above. Each option may be used once, more than once or not at all.

	pH	$p(CO_2)$	$p(O_2)$	Base excess
☐ **12.26**	pH 6.91	$p(CO_2)$ 2.6	$p(O_2)$ 15.7	Base excess −22
☐ **12.27**	pH 7.52	$p(CO_2)$ 2.6	$p(O_2)$ 15.7	Base excess +2
☐ **12.28**	pH 7.37	$p(CO_2)$ 2.6	$p(O_2)$ 9.4	Base excess +2
☐ **12.29**	pH 7.21	$p(CO_2)$ 7.4	$p(O_2)$ 8.4	Base excess +8
Normal values				
	pH 7.36–7.44	$p(CO_2)$ 4.7–5.9 kPa	$p(O_2)$ 11–13 kPa	Base excess −2 to +2mmol/l.

12.30   A 3-year-old girl presents with a 3-month history of recurrent episodes of cough and wheeze. The cough is worse at night. Chest examination is normal between episodes of wheeze, but there is prolonged expiratory wheeze during an episode.

Which one of the following is the most appropriate management?

- [ ] **A**   Arrange chest X-ray
- [ ] **B**   Full blood count
- [ ] **C**   Treat with a course of antibiotics
- [ ] **D**   Trial of antihistaminics
- [ ] **E**   Trial of bronchodilators

12.31   A 60-year-old smoker who was made redundant from his coal mining job in the 1980s presents with exertional dyspnoea and cough. He has a mixed restrictive and obstructive pattern on spirometry. The chest X-ray shows round fibrotic masses in the upper lobes.

Select from the list below the single most likely diagnosis.

- [ ] **A**   Byssinosis
- [ ] **B**   Chronic obstructive pulmonary disease
- [ ] **C**   Lung cancer
- [ ] **D**   Pneumoconiosis
- [ ] **E**   Siderosis

12.32 A 3-year-old boy has had a chronic cough for 3 months. He has had several chest infections and has required several courses of antibiotics. On examination a monophonic wheeze is heard in the right lower lung field. He is systemically well.

Select the single most likely diagnosis from the list below.

☐ **A** Asthma
☐ **B** Croup
☐ **C** Cystic fibrosis
☐ **D** Inhaled foreign body
☐ **E** Whooping cough

12.33 Nebulisers are widely used in both adult and paediatric practice.

Choose the most accurate option from the list below regarding indications for their use.

☐ **A** To deliver an antibiotic (such as colistin) to a patient with chronic purulent infection (as in cystic fibrosis or bronchiectasis)
☐ **B** To deliver a β-agonist to a patient with an acute exacerbation of asthma or COPD
☐ **C** To deliver budesonide to a child with severe croup
☐ **D** All of these
☐ **E** None of these

12.34 Spacer devices remove the need for co-ordination between actuation of a pressurised metered-dose inhaler and inhalation.

Select from the list below the single false statement relating to the use of spacer devices.

☐ **A** A larger proportion of drug particles are deposited in the lungs

☐ **B** Larger spacers are more effective than smaller ones

☐ **C** Patients should inhale as soon as possible after actuation

☐ **D** The full dose of the drug should be deposited in the spacer before inhalation

☐ **E** Tidal breathing is as effective as single breaths

ANSWERS

THEME: SPIROMETRY

Spirometry (meaning the measuring of breath) is the most common of the pulmonary function tests (PFTs). Specifically it measures the amount (volume) and speed (flow) of air that can be inhaled and exhaled. Spirometry is an important tool for assessing conditions such as asthma, pulmonary fibrosis, cystic fibrosis, and COPD. Normal readings in spirometry vary, depending on age, size, and sex.

12.1   B   FEV$_1$

The forced expiratory volume in one second (FEV$_1$) is the amount of air blown out within one second. With normal lungs and airways one can normally blow out most of the air from the lungs within one second. If airways are narrowed, then the amount of air that can be blown out quickly is reduced. So, the FEV$_1$ is reduced and the ratio FEV$_1$/FVC (forced vital capacity) is lower than normal. As a rule, one is likely to have a disease that causes narrowed airways if:

- FEV$_1$ is less than 80% of the predicted value for age, sex and size, or

- FEV$_1$/FVC ratio is 0.7 or less.

12.2   D   FVC

The forced vital capacity (FVC) is the total amount of air that can be blown out in one breath. With narrowed airways, the total capacity of the lungs is often normal or only slightly reduced. So, with an obstructive pattern the FVC is often normal or near normal. With a restrictive lung disease the FVC is less than the predicted value for age, sex and size. This is caused by various conditions that affect the lung tissue itself, or affect the capacity of the lungs to expand and hold a normal amount of air (eg conditions that cause fibrosis or scarring of the lung such as pneumoconiosis or a physical deformity that restricts the expansion of the lungs).

12.3   C   FEV$_1$/FVC

The FEV$_1$ is also reduced in restrictive lung disease but this is in proportion to the reduced FVC. So, with a restrictive pattern the ratio of FEV$_1$/FVC is normal.

12.4   E   Reversibility test

Sometimes, to assess the reversibility of a particular condition, a bronchodilator is administered before performing another round of tests for comparison. This is commonly referred to as a reversibility test and is an important part in distinguishing asthma from COPD.

THEME: MANAGEMENT OF CHRONIC OBSTRUCTIVE PULMONARY DISEASE

12.5   C   Influenza vaccine

There have been only a limited number of studies performed, but it does appear that inactivated vaccine reduces exacerbations in COPD patients.[1] Clinical and laboratory studies have suggested that the currently approved vaccine is less effective in the population of COPD patients than in healthier patients, and to date no randomised-controlled trial of pneumococcal vaccination for COPD patients has demonstrated any beneficial effect.[2]

12.6   A   Amoxicillin

Antibiotics are not indicated except for the treatment of infectious exacerbations and other bacterial infections.[3]

12.7   B   Beclometasone inhaler

Inhaled glucocorticosteroids are recommended for regular use in those in whom the FEV_1 is < 50% (severe COPD) and who have frequent exacerbations (eg three in the last 3 years). Prolonged treatment may relieve symptoms but does not alter the long-term decline in FEV_1.[3]

12.8   H   Tiotropium

Bronchodilaters are the mainstay of symptom management in COPD. When symptoms are persistent they can be given regularly. Regular treatment with long-acting bronchodilators is more effective and convenient than short-acting ones but it is more expensive. The choice is between β_2-agonists (salbutamol, terbutaline, salmeterol), anticholinergics (ipratropium, tiotropium) and methylxanthines (theophylline). Combining drugs with different mechanisms and duration of action may increase the bronchodilation. Theophylline is effective in COPD but is potentially toxic and inhaled bronchodilators are usually preferred. Regular nebulised bronchodilator for stable patients is not appropriate unless it has been shown to be better than conventional doses of a metered dose inhaler.[3]

12.9   D   Oxygen (regular)

Long-term oxygen therapy (LTOT) is indicated in patients with PaO_2 (partial pressure of oxygen in arterial blood) < 7.3kPa when stable, or 7.3–8kPa when stable and one of secondary polycythaemia, nocturnal hypoxaemia, peripheral oedema or pulmonary hypertension. Patients should breathe supplemental oxygen for at least 15 hours a day. The need for oxygen therapy should be assessed in patients with:

- severe airflow obstruction (FEV_1 < 30% predicted)

- cyanosis

- polycythaemia

- peripheral oedema

CHAPTER 12 ANSWERS

- raised jugular venous pressure or

- oxygen saturations less than or equal to 92% breathing air.

Consider assessment for patients with moderate airflow obstruction (FEV$_1$ 30–49% predicted). Practices should have a pulse oximeter to ensure all patients needing LTOT are identified. Oxygen concentrators should be used to provide the fixed supply at home for long-term oxygen therapy.[4] Evidence suggests that domiciliary oxygen improves survival compared with no domiciliary oxygen but not in patients with mild hypoxaemia.[5]

THEME: MANAGEMENT OF ADULT ASTHMA

These answers are based on recommendations of the British Thoracic Society and Scottish Intercollegiate Guidelines Network.[6]

12.10   A   Beclometasone 400µg/day

A stepwise approach is recommended for the management of chronic asthma. This involves stepping up treatment when symptoms are not controlled as well as stepping down when a patient is relatively symptom free.

12.11   B   Beclometasone 800µg/day

Step 1 is the introduction of a short acting bronchodilator with the addition of low dose inhaled corticosteroids as step 2. Step 3 involves the addition of a long-acting β-agonist and, if that combination does not improve the asthma adequately, the inhaled corticosteroid can be increased.

12.12   E   Montelukast 10mg/day

Persistent poor control at step 3 involves the introduction of high dose inhaled cortocosteroids, eg beclometasone 2000 µg/day (step 4). If control is still unsatisfactory a fourth drug (eg leukotriene antagonist, slow-release theophylline, or a β$_2$-agonist tablet is added).

12.13   F   Prednisolone 5mg daily

This patient seems to be having maximum step 4 therapy. Presumably compliance and inhaler technique are good. Step 5 involves the addition of a daily steroid tablet using the lowest dose to provide adequate control. Presumably several short rescue courses of high dose steroids will have already been used in the exacerbations. The high dose of inhaled corticosteroids should be continued. Referral to a chest physician should be considered.

12.14   H   Salbutamol 200µg as required

Presumably this is mild seasonal asthma only and a short acting β_2- agonist for immediate relief is all that is required as long as the pattern of asthma remains the same.

12.15   H   Salbutamol 200µg as required

The description is that of acute severe asthma (respiration > 25 breaths/minute, pulse > 110 beats/minute, inability to complete sentence in one breath). In this case 'as required' for the salbutamol means 4–6 puffs, each inhaled separately via a large-volume spacer. The dose can be repeated every 10–20 minutes. Salbutamol via a nebuliser (oxygen driven if available) is an alternative. If signs of acute asthma continue then urgent hospital admission is needed. While the ambulance is coming the nebulised β_2-agonist can be repeated along with nebulised ipratropium 500µg. If, however, the symptoms settle with the initial management, then a rescue course of prednisolone should be prescribed and the overall management of the asthma reviewed.

THEME: DIAGNOSIS OF RESPIRATORY DISORDERS

12.16   H   Spontaneous pneumothorax

Spontaneous pneumothoraces tend to occur in young people with a tall stature. The reason for this is not known. It is thought that these people may have subtle abnormalities in connective tissue. Some spontaneous pneumothoraces, however, are the result of blister-like structures on the surface of the lung, which rupture allowing the escape of air into the pleural cavity. Sometimes tissue forms a one-way valve that allows air to enter the pleural cavity from the lung but not to escape. Pressure builds up with every breath leading to a tension pneumothorax. In addition to severe shortness of breath there may be circulatory collapse. This condition requires urgent intervention. Treatment involves the insertion of a chest tube.

12.17   E   Pleural effusion

Pleural effusion is an accumulation of fluid in the pleural cavity. Causes include heart failure, malignancy and infections. In this case the subacute onset and weight loss would make malignancy, particularly lung cancer, a likely cause.

12.18   C   Extrinsic allergic alveolitis

The patient has the variety of extrinsic allergic alveolitis known as farmer's lung. Spores from two types of bacteria, *Micropolyspora faeni* and *Thermoactinomyces vulgaris*, and certain types of moulds called aspergillus are the major causes of farmer's lung. Where crops are harvested in wet or rainy weather they usually undergo self-heating while in storage. When this happens, heat-tolerating bacteria and moulds grow rapidly and cause spoilage. As spoiled hay dries, it darkens, crumbles easily, and is extremely dusty. This dust that contains bacteria and mould spores is extremely fine. More modern methods such as the use of silage have diminished the farmer's lung problem. This man presumably buys in fodder for his horses and is experiencing acute attacks after opening up new batches of mouldy hay. In the acute form, symptoms may completely resolve after exposure is removed.

12.19 A Bronchiectasis

Bronchiectasis causes localised, irreversible dilatation of part of the bronchial tree. Involved bronchi are dilated, inflamed, and easily collapsible, resulting in airflow obstruction and impaired clearance of secretions. The cause is often not clear and no cause can be found in over half of cases. Cystic fibrosis, inhaled foreign body or infections such as tuberculosis, whooping cough, measles or pneumonia may be responsible. Diagnosis requires CT scanning. Treatment includes the prolonged usage of antibiotics to treat infections and the elimination of accumulated sputum with postural drainage and chest physiotherapy.

12.20 G Sarcoidosis

The combination of erythema nodosum, bilateral hilar lymphadenopathy and arthralgia is called Löfgren syndrome. This syndrome has a relatively good prognosis. Sarcoidosis is a multisystem disease and can affect many organs. In the lungs it can lead to a restrictive pattern of disease with infiltrates and fibrosis.

THEME: PNEUMONIA

12.21 C *Legionella pneumophila*

A strong presumptive diagnosis of legionella is possible in the majority of patients when three of the following four features are present: a prodromal viral illness; a dry cough, confusion or diarrhoea; lymphopenia without marked leucocytosis; and hyponatraemia.

12.22 B *Klebsiella pneumoniae*

Pneumonia occurs in elderly patients who have a pre-existing co-morbidity such as diabetes and alcoholism. Upper lobe cavitating lesions are common with bulging of the fissures. This organism can be found in sputum and in blood cultures.

CHAPTER 12 ANSWERS

12.23 F *Pseudomonas aeruginosa*

The presence of this organism correlates with a worsening clinical condition and higher mortality in patients with cystic fibrosis. It is important to culture the sputum, as this organism is resistant to most of the common antibiotics used to treat pneumonia.

12.24 D *Mycoplasma pneumoniae*

Infection with this organism may result in cough and dramatic X-ray appearances, which may last for weeks. Patients can have a relapse. Extrapulmonary complications such as pericarditis, haemolytic anaemia, Stevens–Johnson syndrome and neurological problems are rare. Exanthems can also occur.

12.25 E *Pneumocystis jiroveci* (formerly known as *Pneumocystis carinii*)

In contrast to infection with mycoplasma, the clinical features of *Pneumocystis jiroveci* pneumonia are far worse than the radiological appearances. In 90% of cases the diagnosis can be made by using indirect immunofluorescence with monoclonal antibodies to stain sputum.

THEME: BLOOD GAS ANALYSIS

12.26 A Diabetes

A base excess more negative than –2 indicates metabolic acidosis as in this case. A base excess more positive than +2 indicates metabolic alkalosis. This patient is hyperventilating to compensate for the metabolic acidosis. Diabetic ketoacidosis would be the commonest cause.

12.27   E   Primary hyperventilation

This patient is also hyperventilating, which has pushed the blood oxygen above normal and made him mildly alkalotic. There is no hypoxia or metabolic acidosis so no evident reason for the hyperventilation.

12.28   F   Pulmonary embolism

This patient is also hyperventilating but is still hypoxic. This implies a problem with gas exchange in the lungs and an increased ventilation/perfusion ratio mismatch. Pneumonia would be a common cause, but a normal chest X-ray would make pulmonary embolism the likely cause.

12.29   G   Severe asthma

In a moderate asthma attack, the carbon dioxide is low as the patient hyperventilates; as the patient deteriorates and tires the carbon dioxide becomes normal and then raised. This patient is in danger of respiratory arrest.

12.30   E   Trial of bronchodilators

Usually the diagnosis of asthma is clear from the history and examination (including lung function testing), and investigation is not needed. Although a chest X-ray will often show hyperinflation, it will rarely influence management (but an X-ray is helpful for excluding congenital anomalies). Children over the age of 5 years can use a peak-flow meter, but under this age it is difficult to make a definitive diagnosis and often a trial of inhalers is used.

12.31   D   Pneumoconiosis

Pneumoconiosis defines the process of accumulation of dust (often related to occupational exposure) in the lungs, which is permanent and may result in progressive tissue reaction. The condition may progress for many years after initial exposure, and may present with symptoms only after the exposure has ceased. A coal miner would have carbon deposits and a stonemason silicon (silicosis). Siderosis is caused by reaction to iron dust. The chest X-ray findings are vastly out of proportion to the symptoms. Byssinosis is an allergic reaction to cotton dust. The chest X-ray is generally normal. The symptoms are classically worst on Mondays, wane through the week and disappear when away from work.

12.32   D   Inhaled foreign body

Monophonic wheeze is often only heard in one area of the chest. It is produced by partial obstruction of one of the larger airways, either by tumour or inhaled foreign body. Characteristically it is of a single pitch and is often louder in expiration. Polyphonic wheeze is characteristic of small airway obstruction as in asthma or COPD. It is usually heard throughout the lung fields and is characteristically louder in expiration. It is called polyphonic as there are many notes of different pitch, rather like a chord played on a church organ.

Stridor is a harsh noise, classically worse in inspiration and is caused by partial obstruction of the upper airway. It is often associated with features of respiratory distress. Causes of stridor include infective and inflammatory swelling of the upper airway and larynx (as in croup), inhaled foreign bodies and tumours of the upper airway.

In the established coughing phase of whooping cough the patient repeatedly coughs. The face often goes red and the body becomes tense. Eventually, there is a desperate attempt to breathe in, which may cause a 'whooping' sound.

12.33   D   All of these[7]

A nebuliser converts a solution of a drug into an aerosol for inhalation. It is used to deliver a higher dose of drug than is usual with standard inhaler devices. The British Thoracic Society has issued guidelines for best practice in the use of nebulisers.[7]

12.34   D   The full dose of the drug should be deposited in the spacer before inhalation

Patients should inhale as soon as possible after actuation because the drug aerosol is very short lived. If a larger dose of drug requires more than one actuation then there should be a separate inhalation for each actuation rather than waiting for the full dose to be deposited before inhaling.[8]

REFERENCES

1. Poole PJ, Chacko E, Wood-Baker RWB, Cates CJ. *Influenza vaccine for patients with chronic obstructive pulmonary disease. Cochrane Database of Systematic Reviews* 2000, Issue 4. Art. No.: CD002733. DOI: 10.1002/14651858.CD002733.pub2

2. Schenkein JG, Nahm MH, Dransfield MT. Pneumococcal Vaccination for Patients with COPD: Current Practice and Future Directions. *Chest.* 2008; 133: 767-774.

3. *Global initiative for chronic obstructive lung disease. Pocket Guide to COPD Diagnosis, Management, and Prevention.* (homepage on the Internet), July 2003 (updated 2007, cited 2008 May 5). Available from http://www.goldcopd.com/Guidelineitem.asp?l1=2&l2=1&intId=1116

4. National Institute for Health and Clinical Excellence. *Chronic obstructive pulmonary disease: Quick reference guide.* (homepage on the Internet), February 2004 (cited 2008 May 5). Available from http://www.nice.org.uk/guidance/CG12/?c=91527

5. Crockett AJ, Moss JR, Cranston JM, et al. *Domiciliary oxygen in chronic obstructive pulmonary disease.* In: The Cochrane Library, Issue 1, 2005. Oxford: Update Software. Search date 2000; primary source Cochrane Airways Group Register.

6. British Thoracic Society and Scottish Intercollegiate Guidelines Network. *British Guideline on the Management of Asthma* (homepage on the Internet), February 2003 (updated July 2007; cited 2008 April 28). Available from http://www.sign.ac.uk/guidelines/fulltext/63/index.html

7. British Thoracic Society. *Nebuliser Treatment Best Practice Guideline* (homepage on the Internet), 1997 (cited 2008 May 10). Available from http://www.brit-thoracic.org.uk/ClinicalInformation/NebuliserTreatmentBestPractice/tabid/101/Default.aspx

8. *Peak flow meters, inhaler devices and nebulisers.* 3.1.5. British National Formulary; 55; 2008.

CHAPTER 12 ANSWERS

Mock Exam

Chapter 13
Clinical Problem Solving – Example Test Paper

QUESTIONS

Total time allowed is 75 minutes

THEME: HYPERTENSION TREATMENT

Options

A Amlodipine

B Atenolol

C Bendroflumethiazide

D Doxazosin

E Lisinopril

F Losartan

G Methyl dopa

H Moxonidine

For each of the hypertensive patients below, choose the single most likely antihypertensive medication from the list of options above. Each option may be used once, more than once or not at all.

☐ **13.1** A 60-year-old man with diabetes who is already taking an angiotensin-converting enzyme (ACE) inhibitor.

☐ **13.2** A 42-year-old African Caribbean woman with hypertension not controlled by bendroflumethiazide.

☐ **13.3** A 72-year-old man with poorly controlled hypertension who has recently developed angina.

☐ **13.4** A 41-year-old-woman with chronic obstructive pulmonary disease who is taking ramipril and bendroflumethiazide but has developed a persistent dry cough, which does not seem to be related to her airways disease.

☐ **13.5** A 35-year-old pregnant woman whose blood pressure is 170/110mmHg in the mid-trimester.

THEME: INFECTIOUS DISEASES IN CHILDHOOD

Options

A Intravenous aciclovir

B Intravenous antibiotic

C Oral aciclovir

D Oral antibiotic

E Symptomatic relief (antipyretics and/or analgesics)

F Topical aciclovir

G Topical antibiotic

For each of the patients below, choose the single most appropriate management option from the list of options above. Each option may be used once, more than once or not at all.

☐ **13.6** A 14-year-old girl has a 10-day history of fever and malaise. On examination there is prominent cervical lymphadenopathy.

☐ **13.7** A previously well 4-year-old girl has a fever and vesicular rash. It started as a papular rash on the trunk and spread peripherally with new spots appearing in crops.

☐ **13.8** A 10-month-old baby boy has fever and a widespread tender erythematous rash. The infant looks unwell and the skin is peeling in places.

☐ **13.9** A 3-year-old girl has multiple painful erosions on the mucosa of the mouth and tongue with erythema and swelling of the gums.

☐ **13.10** A 6-month-old baby boy has bilateral red eyes. There is a creamy sticky exudate in both eyes.

THEME: CHEST PAIN

Options

A Acute angina

B Bronchial carcinoma

C Chest infection

D Musculoskeletal pain

E Myocardial infarction

F Oesophageal reflux

G Pulmonary embolism

H Spontaneous pneumothorax

I Unstable angina

For each of the patients below, choose the single most likely diagnosis from the list of options above. Each option may be used once, more than once or not at all.

☐ **13.11** A 62-year-old woman with chronic obstructive pulmonary disease presents with increasing wheeze and cough. Her inhalers are not working well and she has been coughing up purulent sputum. Her chest pain is much worse on deep inspiration and she has a slight fever.

☐ **13.12** A 32-year-old woman presents with worsening shortness of breath and pain on deep inspiration. She had her first baby 2 weeks ago and is usually fit and well.

☐ **13.13** A 52-year-old builder smokes 25 cigarettes a day. He has worsening left-sided chest pain which does not radiate and he can point one finger to the site of the pain. It has been present for 2 days and he is usually fit and well.

CHAPTER 13 QUESTIONS

☐ **13.14** A 73-year-old woman has coronary heart disease. She takes aspirin, atenolol and ramipril. The past 3 nights she has been awoken in the night with left-sided chest pain radiating down her left arm. She has tried her glyceryl trinitrate spray but without effect, the pain passing off eventually after about half an hour.

☐ **13.15** A 56-year-old bricklayer presents with central chest pain for 2 days. It is not related to exertion. He has been working overtime recently and taking regular ibuprofen for a sprained wrist.

THEME: FACIAL RASHES

Options

A	Acne vulgaris	F	Rosacea
B	Actinic keratoses	G	Seborrhoeic eczema
C	Erysipelas	H	Sunburn
D	Perioral dermatitis	I	Systemic lupus erythematosus
E	Psoriasis		

For each of the patients below, choose the single most likely diagnosis from the list of options above. Each option may be used once, more than once or not at all.

☐ **13.16** A 13-year-old girl has papules and comedones on her chin and forehead. She cleanses her face twice a day. She has recently started her periods.

☐ **13.17** A 70-year-old man has erythematous macules and papules with coarse adherent scale on his forehead and bald scalp. Many of the lesions have become confluent.

☐ **13.18** A 30-year-old woman has papules and erythema around the mouth and on her chin. Her son's topical steroid helped but the rash became much worse when she stopped using it.

☐ **13.19** A 65-year-old woman has a persistent erythematous eruption on her forehead and cheeks. It has become much worse after her summer holiday to Italy. There are a few pustules within it.

☐ **13.20** A 45-year-old man has had dandruff for many years. He has greasy, red and scaly skin on his central face and forehead. The sides of his nose down to the outer ends of his mouth are also affected.

CHAPTER 13 QUESTIONS

THEME: MACROSCOPIC HAEMATURIA

Options

A   Bladder cancer

B   Glomerulonephritis

C   Haemorrhagic cystitis (urinary infection)

D   Prostate cancer

E   Prostatitis

F   Renal cancer

G   Renal cyst

H   Schistosomiasis

I   Sickle cell disease

J   Ureteric calculus

For each of the patients below, choose the single most likely diagnosis from the list of options above. Each option may be used once, more than once or not at all.

☐ **13.21** A partially sighted 80-year-old woman has a fractured humerus after a trivial injury. She is catheterised and found to have macroscopic haematuria.

☐ **13.22** A 50-year-old man has terminal uralgia, frequency and haematuria. Urine culture does not reveal any organisms.

☐ **13.23** A 20-year-old male visitor from Egypt has severe frequency and dysuria and has seen blood in his urine.

☐ **13.24** A 70-year-old woman has recently started taking warfarin for atrial fibrillation. She feels well but notices blood in her urine.

☐ **13.25** A 90-year-old woman in a nursing home uses pads for urinary incontinence. She is already taking antibiotics for a urinary infection, has new-onset confusion and now frank haematuria.

CHAPTER 13 QUESTIONS

THEME: SHORT STATURE IN CHILDREN

Options

A Achondroplasia

B Congenital hypothyroidism

C Down syndrome

D Growth hormone deficiency

E Klinefelter syndrome

F Noonan syndrome

G Russell–Silver syndrome

H Turner syndrome

For each of the children below, choose the most likely cause of short stature from the list of options above. Each option may be used once, more than once or not at all.

☐ **13.26** A child with an abnormally sized head and predominant shortening of the proximal upper and lower limbs.

☐ **13.27** A 6-year-old boy with webbing of the neck, cubitus valgus and congenital heart disease.

☐ **13.28** A 7-year-old boy previously treated with cranial irradiation for a brain tumour with recurrent episodes of hypoglycaemia.

☐ **13.29** A 2-year-old with poor motor and speech development, large tongue and umbilical hernia.

CHAPTER 13 QUESTIONS

THEME: CAUSES OF A NON-BLANCHING RASH

Options

A Acute leukaemia

B Cushing disease

C Fat embolism syndrome

D Haemolytic–uraemic syndrome

E Henoch–Schönlein purpura

F Immune thrombocytopenic purpura

G Meningococcal septicaemia

H Non-accidental injury

For each of the following descriptions, choose the single most likely diagnosis from the list of options above. Each option may be used once, more than once or not at all.

☐ **13.30** A child with malaise and a mild fever presents with a purpuric rash on the buttocks and legs. Otherwise he is well.

☐ **13.31** Following a recent upper respiratory tract infection, a previously well child has started to bruise easily. The platelet count is 10 x 10^9/l.

☐ **13.32** A child presents with four lines of purpura along the outer thigh. The platelet count is 200 x 10^9/l.

☐ **13.33** A very sick child with high fever, has a purpuric rash on the limbs and a prolonged capillary refill time.

☐ **13.34** A 6-year-old child has developed widespread petechiae and is pale. She has been unwell for a few weeks with recurrent infections.

THEME: INVESTIGATIONS OF PRURITUS VULVAE

Options

A Creatinine clearance

B Glucose tolerance test

C High vaginal swab

D Vulval biopsy

E None of the above

For each presentation of pruritus vulvae below, choose the single most appropriate investigation from the list above. Each option may be used once, more than once or not at all.

☐ **13.35 A woman with associated history of vaginal discharge.**

☐ **13.36 A woman with a history of postmenopausal bleeding.**

☐ **13.37 This investigation is unnecessary in pruritus vulvae.**

☐ **13.38 A 45-year-old woman with associated vulval ulceration.**

☐ **13.39 In a 50-year-old obese woman with features of candidiasis.**

CHAPTER 13 QUESTIONS

THEME: CAUSES OF CLUBBING

Options

A Axillary artery aneurysm

B Bronchiectasis

C Coeliac disease

D Crohn disease

E Cyanotic congenital heart disease

F Cystic fibrosis

G Fibrosing alveolitis

H Hepatic cirrhosis

I Hyperthyroidism

J Infective endocarditis

K Mesothelioma

L Squamous cell lung cancer

For each patient below, choose the most likely cause of clubbing from the list of options above. Each option may be used once, more than once or not at all.

☐ **13.40** A 74-year-old man has fever and breathlessness. He recently had a transurethral resection of the prostate but was otherwise well until 3 weeks ago. His temperature is 37.7°C, his pulse is 96/min and regular, and his blood pressure is 180/80mmHg. He has an early diastolic murmur. His chest is clear. Blood is seen on urine dipstick test. He has evidence of early clubbing.

☐ **13.41** A 27-year-old woman has recurrent chest infections and has a chronic productive cough. She remembers having had whooping cough as a child. She is not febrile or cyanosed but has marked clubbing. She has widespread crackles and a wheeze which do not clear with coughing.

☐ **13.42** A 68-year-old man has a 3-month history of cough and weight loss. He is cachectic and has a hyperexpanded, quiet chest with no abnormal breath sounds heard. He has left-sided ptosis and bilateral clubbing. He recently stopped smoking and gives a history of asbestos exposure.

☐ **13.43** A 15-year-old boy is under investigation for weight loss. He has intermittent abdominal pain and diarrhoea. His stools are often pale and hard to flush away. He is thin and pale-skinned with fair hair but with no specific abnormalities apart from clubbing.

☐ **13.44** A 53-year-old man has clubbing in the left hand only. He has hypertension and angina, with three-vessel coronary disease shown on angiography 2 years ago. His hypertension and angina are well controlled.

THEME: COMMON PRESENTATIONS IN SPORTSMEN/WOMEN

Options

A Anterior knee pain

B Bucket handle meniscus tear

C Carpal tunnel syndrome

D Lateral epicondylitis

E Plantar fasciitis

F Prepatellar bursitis

G Pulled elbow

H Shin splints

I Trochanteric bursitis

J Ulnar collateral ligament rupture

For each of the presentations below, choose the single most appropriate answer from the list above. Each option may be used once, more than once or not at all.

☐ **13.45** A skier consults after a fall in which he was not seriously injured. He fell doing slalom while holding his ski poles and now has pain.

☐ **13.46** An amateur runner is trying to train for the London Marathon.

☐ **13.47** A professional violin player presents with pain during rehearsals.

☐ **13.48** A footballer has fallen during a tackle.

☐ **13.49** A female competitive rower complains of pain.

THEME: HEADACHE

Options

A Brain tumour
B Cluster headache
C Migraine
D Subarachnoid haemorrhage
E Temporal arteritis
F Tension headache
E Trigeminal neuralgia

For each of the patients below, choose the single most likely diagnosis from the list of options above. Each option may be used once, more than once or not at all.

☐ **13.50** A 33-year-old housewife comes to your surgery complaining of worsening headache over 24 hours. This has been associated with nausea and some photophobia. That morning, before the headache started, she saw some zig-zag lines and felt unwell. She is otherwise well and only takes an oral contraceptive pill.

☐ **13.51** A 42-year-old man complains of recurrent headaches on the left side of his head. The pain comes on very rapidly and sometimes when he has the headache his left eye becomes watery and bloodshot. He is a smoker.

☐ **13.52** A 48-year-old man has a worsening headache at the back of his head. He has recently changed jobs and been under a lot of stress. He says the headache came on suddenly during the night and woke him from his sleep. He also has some photophobia.

☐ **13.53** A 70-year-old man describes a sharp, intermittent pain on the left side of his face. It often comes on when he is shaving or eating. The pain lasts a couple of minutes. He says it is very severe.

☐ **13.54** A 45-year-old nurse complains of worsening headache. She describes it like a band across her forehead, sometimes worse on the left side. It worsens throughout the day. Simple analgesics are ineffective and she is worried she may have a brain tumour.

☐ **13.55** A 67-year-old man complains of a worsening, severe headache which is often aggravated by combing his hair. He has been feeling more tired than usual.

THEME: FAILURE TO CONCEIVE

Options

A Endocervical and high vaginal swab

B Hysterosalpingogram

C Karyotype analysis

D Pelvic ultrasound scan

E Serum luteinising hormone (LH) and follicle-stimulating hormone (FSH)

F Serum prolactin

G Serum testosterone

For each of the scenarios described below, choose the single most appropriate initial investigation from the list of options above. Each option may be used once, more than once or not at all.

☐ **13.56** A 26-year-old has failed to conceive after one year. Her periods are regular. She has normal secondary sexual characteristics. Pelvic examination reveals right adnexal tenderness. She admits to several 'one night stands' in the past although she is currently in a steady relationship.

☐ **13.57** A 30-year-old has been trying to conceive for 18 months. She has irregular periods which can be anything from 2–6 weeks apart, and she also had acne in her early 20s. On examination she is slightly overweight, but there are no other remarkable findings. LH and FSH are within the normal range.

☐ **13.58** A 44-year-old would like to become pregnant. She was recently married and is keen to start a family as quickly as possible. Her periods used to be regular but recently have been more infrequent, at intervals of 6–8 weeks.

☐ **13.59** An 18-year-old woman presents with primary amenorrhoea. She is worried about whether she will ever be able to have children. There is a lack of breast development and other secondary sexual characteristics and she is of short stature.

THEME: COLONIC DISORDERS

Options

A	Carcinoma of the caecum	E	Diverticulitis
B	Carcinoma of the sigmoid colon	F	Haemorrhoids
		G	Irritable bowel syndrome
C	Colonic polyp	H	Sigmoid volvulus
D	Crohn disease	I	Ulcerative colitis

For each patient below, choose the most appropriate diagnosis from the list of options above. Each option may be used once, more than once or not at all.

☐ **13.60** A 72-year-old man presents with increasing tiredness over a 2-year period. He has microcytic anaemia and a mass in the right iliac fossa.

☐ **13.61** A 33-year-old woman consults you regarding symptoms of alternating diarrhoea and constipation associated with cramp-like abdominal pain.

☐ **13.62** A 76-year-old man presents with weight loss, pain on eating and abdominal distension. Plain abdominal X-ray films show the so-called 'coffee bean' sign.

☐ **13.63** An 82-year-old woman presents to the Emergency Department with a distended abdomen. A plain abdominal X-ray film shows gross faecal loading in the colon and gas in the small bowel. The rectum is empty.

☐ **13.64** A 39-year-old woman presents with passage of bloodstained motions and mucus five times a day. Symptoms have persisted for over 1 month and are associated with weight loss. Barium enema shows no evidence of a colonic neoplasm, but a granular mucosa.

THEME: MONITORING OF DRUGS

Options

A Amiodarone

B Azathioprine

C Levodopa

D Lithium

E Phenytoin

F Ramipril

G Simvastatin

H Warfarin

For each monitoring regimen below select the single most likely drug from the list above to which it applies. Each option may be used once, more than once or not at all.

☐ **13.65** Measure blood levels after each change of dose.

☐ **13.66** Do a full blood count weekly for 4 weeks, thereafter every 3 months.

☐ **13.67** Measure serum concentrations every 3 months and thyroid function every 6 months.

☐ **13.68** Measure renal function before starting, after 1 month and yearly during treatment.

THEME: CAUSES OF A SORE MOUTH

Options

A   Antibiotic associated candidosis

B   Burning mouth syndrome

C   Coated tongue

D   Geographic tongue

E   Iron deficiency

F   Lichen planus

G   Oral hairy leucoplakia

H   Squamous cell carcinoma

I   Systemic lupus erythematosus

J   Thrush

K   Trauma

L   Vitamin B_{12} deficiency

For each of the following scenarios, choose the most likely diagnosis from the list of options above. Each option may be used once, more than once or not at all.

☐ **13.69** A 20-year-old woman has become concerned about recurrent episodes of tongue soreness exacerbated by spicy foods. She says that she has seen areas of erythematous smooth red areas on her tongue which seem to move over the weeks.

☐ **13.70** A 65-year-old heavy smoker has had a long-standing increasingly painful ulcer on the lateral border of his tongue. He first noticed the ulcer 3 months ago and he is now having difficulty speaking.

☐ **13.71** A 55-year-old woman with a pruritic skin rash affecting her wrists and shins has also noticed oral soreness. On examination of her mouth there are areas of white striae and ulceration affecting her tongue and buccal mucosa.

☐ **13.72** A 70-year-old woman is found to have a smooth, sore, red tongue with soreness and cracking at the corners of her mouth. She is undergoing investigation for a mass in her right iliac fossa.

☐ **13.73** A 23-year-old man with asthma complains of a sore mouth. On examination he is found to have an inflamed palate with white specks and a smooth red tongue.

THEME: CHILD WITH A PAINFUL LEG

Options

A   Fractured femur
B   Irritable hip
C   Non-accidental injury
D   Osgood–Schlatter disease
E   Osteomyelitis
F   Perthes disease
G   Septic arthritis
H   Shin splints
I   Sickle cell disease
J   Slipped femoral epiphysis

For each of the patients below, choose the single most likely diagnosis from the list of options above. Each option may be used once, more than once or not at all.

☐ **13.74** A 5-year-old boy has a painful limp for a few weeks. Examination reveals limited movement at the hip. X-ray of the hip shows sclerosis of the femoral head. The parents deny any trauma.

☐ **13.75** A 13-year-old boy who is overweight develops hip pain after a minor fall. An X-ray of the hip shows abnormal findings.

☐ **13.76** A 12-year-old child who enjoys sports develops a tender tibial tuberosity.

☐ **13.77** A 6-year-old boy develops a limp after an upper respiratory tract infection. X-rays show normal findings.

☐ **13.78** A 5-month-old girl is brought in to the Emergency Department by her nanny because she has been crying all morning. Her left thigh is swollen. There is no history of trauma.

CHAPTER 13 QUESTIONS

13.79 A 26-year-old woman developed a high fever and vomiting on the third day of her period. She then developed a macular erythematous rash over her face and trunk, associated with confusion, conjunctival suffusion, peripheral oedema and a strawberry-like appearance of her tongue.

Select the single most probable diagnosis from the list below.

- [ ] **A** Stevens–Johnson syndrome
- [ ] **B** Toxic epidermal necrolysis
- [ ] **C** Toxic shock syndrome
- [ ] **D** Typhoid fever
- [ ] **E** Yellow fever

13.80 A 21-year-old woman has several localised papular lesions on her hands and feet. One of the partners in the practice has seen her and diagnosed granuloma annulare.

Select the single most appropriate investigation for this woman from the list below.

- [ ] **A** Fasting blood sugar
- [ ] **B** HbA1c level
- [ ] **C** Skin biopsy
- [ ] **D** Skin scraping for fungal culture
- [ ] **E** Thyroid function tests

13.81   Which one of the following diseases is not notifiable under the Public Health Act 1984 and Public Health Regulations 1988?

- [ ] **A**   Food poisoning
- [ ] **B**   Mumps
- [ ] **C**   Parvovirus infection
- [ ] **D**   Scarlet fever
- [ ] **E**   Whooping cough

13.82   A 52-year-old postmenopausal woman presents with general fatigue. Blood tests show that her serum aminotransferase level is 160 IU/l and alkaline phosphatase level is 185 U/l with bilirubin 35μmol/l. A full blood count shows mild normocytic normochromic anaemia with thrombocytopenia and leucopenia. Liver biopsy shows chronic inflammatory cell infiltrate with lymphocytes, plasma cells and sometimes lymphoid follicles in the portal tracts. (Normal values: bilirubin 3–17μmol/l, alanine aminotransferase 5–35 IU/l, alkaline phosphatase 30–150 U/l. Select the single most probable diagnosis from the list below.

- [ ] **A** α_1-AT deficiency
- [ ] **B**   Autoimmune hepatitis
- [ ] **C**   Chronic hepatitis C infection
- [ ] **D**   Infectious mononucleosis
- [ ] **E**   Non-alcoholic steatohepatitis (NASH)

13.83 **Which of the following is an indication of a severe, life-threatening asthma exacerbation?**

- [ ] **A** Peak expiratory flow rate (PEFR) < 50% best or predicted
- [ ] **B** Reduced response to β_2-agonist inhaler
- [ ] **C** Stridor
- [ ] **D** Tachypnoea > 25 breaths/minute
- [ ] **E** Tachycardia > 100 beats/minute

13.84 **A 45-year-old woman presents with neck and arm pain.**

Which of the following signs if present should lead to prompt neurosurgical referral?

- [ ] **A** Brisk biceps reflex
- [ ] **B** Decreased grip strength
- [ ] **C** Decreased pronator jerk
- [ ] **D** Loss of sensation in the little finger
- [ ] **E** Neck stiffness

13.85 **Which one of the following people has the greatest risk of attempting suicide?**

- [ ] **A** A 17-year-old student who has recently split with her boyfriend
- [ ] **B** A 24-year-old unemployed single man
- [ ] **C** A 34-year-old mother with postnatal depression
- [ ] **D** A 62-year-old widow who has recently been diagnosed with depression
- [ ] **E** A 78-year-old man with exacerbation of his chronic obstructive pulmonary disease

13.86   **Which one of the following is not a risk factor for stroke?**

☐   **A**   Atrial fibrillation
☐   **B**   Diabetes mellitus
☐   **C**   Hypertension
☐   **D**   Hypothyroidism
☐   **E**   Obesity

13.87   A 38-year-old woman, 10 days' post partum, presents with a history of foul-smelling discharge per vagina. She has been passing blood clots per vagina for 24 hours. Her blood pressure is 90/40mmHg, pulse 110 beats/minute, and temperature 38°C. Her uterus is tender on palpation and the fundus reaches the umbilicus.

Select the single most probable diagnosis from the list below.

☐   **A**   Cervical tear
☐   **B**   Menorrhagia
☐   **C**   Pelvic inflammatory disease
☐   **D**   Primary post-partum haemorrhage
☐   **E**   Secondary post-partum haemorrhage

CHAPTER 13 QUESTIONS

13.88   An 18-year-old woman has moderately severe acne vulgaris with a mixture of inflamed papules and pustules and closed and open comedones. She takes a combined oral contraceptive. You decide to treat her with oxytetracycline.

Select from the list below the single correct piece of information.

- [ ] **A**   An additional contraceptive method will need to be used long-term
- [ ] **B**   Comedones are more likely to clear than the inflamed lesions
- [ ] **C**   Rapid improvement can be expected
- [ ] **D**   The dose of the drug is 500mg twice daily
- [ ] **E**   The normal duration of treatment is 3 months

13.89   Which one of the following drugs causes gingival hyperplasia?

- [ ] **A**   Allopurinol
- [ ] **B**   Atenolol
- [ ] **C**   Phenytoin
- [ ] **D**   Ramipril
- [ ] **E**   Sodium valproate

13.90   Which one of the following statements about statins is correct?

- [ ] **A**   All patients with hypertension should be taking a statin
- [ ] **B**   Patients with a 10-year cardiovascular disease risk of more than 20% should receive a statin for primary prevention
- [ ] **C**   Patients with type 2 diabetes should have their cardiovascular risk calculated to assess their need for a statin
- [ ] **D**   Statins are better than fibrates in reducing triglyceride levels
- [ ] **E**   They should be prescribed only for patients with established coronary heart disease

13.91 A 56-year-old man has recently had some blood tests performed by the practice nurse. He comes to see you, worried he may have diabetes because he has been very thirsty and has lost some weight.

Which one of the following results would confirm this diagnosis?

- [ ] **A** Fasting glucose: 6.9mmol/l
- [ ] **B** Fasting glucose: 8.1mmol/l
- [ ] **C** Glucose 1 hour after oral glucose tolerance test: 10.8mmol/l
- [ ] **D** HbA1c: 8.2%
- [ ] **E** Random glucose: 9.2mmol/l

13.92 Which one of the following is not a normal variant in babies?

- [ ] **A** A 12-hour-old baby with jaundice
- [ ] **B** An urticarial looking rash on a 3-day-old baby
- [ ] **C** Blue looking feet in a 1-day-old baby
- [ ] **D** Non-retractile foreskin in a 6-month-old boy
- [ ] **E** Sneezing in a 2-hour-old baby
- [ ] **F** Tiny cream pearls on the hard palate in a newborn baby
- [ ] **G** Very dry skin in a newborn baby born at 42 weeks' gestation

13.93 A 30-year-old mountain biker who frequently competes on forest terrain complains of a flu-like illness, splenomegaly and arthralgia.

Select the single most likely cause from the list below.

- [ ] **A** *Borrelia burgdorferi* infection
- [ ] **B** Fasciolopsiasis
- [ ] **C** Filariasis
- [ ] **D** Giardiasis
- [ ] **E** Toxacariasis

13.94 A 67-year-old woman who consumes a low-fibre diet presents with a short history of lower abdominal pain, more so in the left iliac fossa (LIF), associated with nausea and constipation. She can tolerate oral fluids. On examination you note she looks mildly unwell with a temperature of 37.5°C.

Select from the list below the next most appropriate step in management.

☐ **A** Admit urgently to surgical team for assessment

☐ **B** Arrange a barium enema X-ray

☐ **C** Increase her laxatives and review in 1 week

☐ **D** Prescribe an anti-spasmodic drug

☐ **E** Treat with broad-spectrum antibiotics

13.95 A 68-year-old woman presents to her GP with general symptoms of tiredness, weight loss and sweating during the night. She seems to be generally depressed. Further enquiry reveals she has stiffness and pain in her shoulders and neck, which is worse in the morning and lasts about 30 minutes.

What is the single best investigation for this condition from the list below?

☐ **A** Autoantibody screen

☐ **B** Erythrocyte sedimentation rate (ESR)

☐ **C** Muscle biopsy

☐ **D** Nerve conduction velocity

☐ **E** Temporal artery biopsy

13.96   A 32-year-old man diagnosed as having type 1 diabetes mellitus was started on Mixtard insulin. However, control proved to be a problem, with hypoglycaemia between meals and particularly at night. This was substituted with rapid-acting insulin analogues, but has resulted in erratic morning blood sugar readings.

Which one of the following is the single best management option to overcome this problem?

- [ ] **A**   Add a sulphonylurea
- [ ] **B**   Add insulin glargine
- [ ] **C**   Add the new class of insulin secretagogues – repaglinide
- [ ] **D**   Add twice daily medium-acting insulin
- [ ] **E**   Adjust the dose of a rapid-acting insulin according to blood glucose results

13.97   A 62-year-old politician has been finding it increasingly difficult to remember all the information at his daily party meetings. This has been followed by a decline in language function: he finds it difficult to remember the names of his colleagues, and planning, organising and abstracting have also become difficult. Now, at times, he also becomes agitated and aggressive. There is a history of similar deterioration of function in the family.

Select the single most likely diagnosis from the list below.

- [ ] **A**   Alzheimer disease
- [ ] **B**   Creutzfeldt–Jakob disease
- [ ] **C**   Lewy body dementia
- [ ] **D**   Multi-infarct dementia
- [ ] **E**   Parkinson's disease

13.98 A 20-week pregnant woman has a recent history of indirect exposure to chickenpox as one of her neighbour's children has chickenpox. The patient is not sure whether she had chickenpox as a child.

Select the single best management for this patient from the list below.

☐ **A** Aciclovir

☐ **B** Check for serum varicella zoster IgG

☐ **C** Immunoglobulins and aciclovir

☐ **D** Termination of pregnancy

☐ **E** Varicella zoster vaccination

13.99 Which one of the following is not a cause of reduced fertility in men?

☐ **A** Past history of testicular torsion

☐ **B** Peyronie disease

☐ **C** Previous mumps infection

☐ **D** Smoking

☐ **E** Undescended testicle

13.100 A 24-year-old man presents with right earache and deafness that has worsened over 24 hours. His ear has started discharging and the pain has improved.

Select the single most likely diagnosis from the list below.

☐ **A** Acute otitis externa

☐ **B** Acute otitis media

☐ **C** Chronic suppurative otitis media

☐ **D** Glue ear

☐ **E** Wax

ANSWERS

THEME: HYPERTENSION TREATMENT

13.1   A   Amlodipine

All patients with diabetes and hypertension should be taking an ACE inhibitor, unless it is contraindicated. β-Blockers should not be used to treat hypertension in diabetic patients (unless they are needed for coronary heart disease). Diuretics are sometimes used for diabetic patients but would not be used first or even second line.[1]

13.2   E   Lisinopril

The National Institute for Health and Clinical Excellence (NICE) guidelines[1] state that calicum channel blockers or thiazide diuretics should be used first line for black patients at any age. An ACE inhibitor should be added to the initial therapy if the blood pressure is not controlled.

13.3   B   Atenolol

β-blockers are still used for coronary heart disease and would be very suitable for this patient. β-blockers are no longer used as first line treatment as studies have shown that they are less effective at reducing cardiovascular events.[2]

13.4   F   Losartan

Angiotensin-II receptor blockers would be suitable for this woman as it appears she has developed an ACE-related cough. She should be reviewed to ensure her cough improves on stopping the ACE inhibitor. Around 10% of patients taking ACE inhibitors develop an ACE inhibitor cough.

13.5   G   Methyl dopa

Sustained hypertension greater than 160/100mmHg in pregnancy is usually an indication for treatment. Hypertension increases the risk of pre-eclampsia and placental abruption. The centrally acting agent methyl dopa is the drug of choice. Labetalol, nifedipine and hydralazine are also sometimes used.

THEME: INFECTIOUS DISEASES IN CHILDHOOD

13.6   E   Symptomatic relief (antipyretics and/or analgesics)

This is likely to be infectious mononucleosis, most commonly caused by the Epstein–Barr virus. It typically infects older children and is spread via oral secretions. Other features include tonsillitis/pharyngitis, splenomegaly, hepatomegaly, jaundice, maculopapular rash. Symptoms may persist for some months but treatment is symptomatic.

13.7   E   Symptomatic relief (antipyretics and/or analgesics)

This is most likely varicella zoster infection (chickenpox). It is spread is by the respiratory route and has a 14-day incubation period. Most patients will become symptomatic with the infection. It is highly infectious. Crops of new spots occur for typically 3–5 days then the lesions crust over. Uncomplicated infection in a child who is not immunocompromised requires only symptomatic treatment.

13.8   B   Intravenous antibiotic

This is scalded skin syndrome – a staphylococcal skin infection. Typically the skin is red and tender and areas of epidermis may separate on gentle pressure (Nikolsky sign). Intravenous antibiotics are required as this is a serious infection.

13.9   C   Oral aciclovir

This is primary herpes simplex infection. The *British National Formulary*[3] recommends a soft diet, adequate fluid, analgesia, benzydamine rinse or spray and the use of chlorhexidine mouthwash. In the case of severe herpes stomatitis, systemic aciclovir is required. There is no suggestion that this child is immunocompromised so the oral route seems appropriate.

13.10   G   Topical antibiotic

This is likely to be conjunctivitis. The conjunctiva will be red and inflamed. It can be allergic, bacterial or viral in nature. The presence of a purulent discharge, however, suggests a bacterial origin, and topical antibiotic drops or ointment will be appropriate.

THEME: CHEST PAIN

13.11   C   Chest infection

It is very likely that this woman has a chest infection. She is more prone to chest infections as she has chronic obstructive pulmonary disease. She has some pleuritic chest pain which is classically worse on deep inspiration. She should be treated with antibiotics and anti-inflammatory analgesics.

13.12   G   Pulmonary embolism

Pulmonary embolism is the most likely diagnosis for this woman. There is an increased risk of venous thromboembolism post partum. Her legs should be examined for any clinical signs of deep vein thrombosis and she should be admitted to hospital.

13.13   D   Musculoskeletal pain

This is the most likely diagnosis as the history is not typical for angina. However, it is important to exclude angina as, being a smoker, he is at an increased risk of coronary heart disease. His risk factors for coronary heart disease should be addressed in this consultation.

13.14   I   Unstable angina

This woman has unstable angina as it is occurring at rest. She is at a high risk of having another myocardial infarction and should be admitted to hospital.

13.15   F   Oesophageal reflux

It is most likely that the anti-inflammatory drug he is taking for his wrist has caused some gastric irritation leading to indigestion and reflux symptoms. He should stop taking ibuprofen.

THEME: FACIAL RASHES

13.16   A   Acne vulgaris

Acne is very common – affecting around 50% of teenagers with varying severity. Despite various beliefs, acne is not usually worsened by eating chocolate. Acne usually worsens during puberty.

13.17   B   Actinic keratoses

Actinic keratoses are due to prolonged and repeated solar exposure and hence are more common on the face and scalp. The scale is quite adherent and only removed with difficulty and pain. The skin is rough like sandpaper. Highly hypertrophic lesions and cutaneous horns may require biopsy to exclude squamous cell carcinoma.

13.18   D   Perioral dermatitis

This is most likely to be perioral dermatitis. Topical steroids exacerbate the condition. Treatment is with topical or systemic antibiotics (oxytetracycline or erythromycin for 4 weeks or longer).

13.19   F   Rosacea

Rosacea is the most likely diagnosis. It can often be confused with acne vulgaris in which there are comedones, a wider distribution and improvement with sunlight. Topical steroids should be avoided in patients with rosacea because they exacerbate the condition. Sunlight and alcohol also can make it worse.

13.20   G   Seborrhoeic eczema

Skin infection by yeast called *Pityrosporum* is thought to play a part in seborrhoeic eczema. Anti-yeast treatment can therefore be effective, although it usually needs to be repeated periodically. A mixture of antifungal cream and mild steroid (1% hydrocortisone) is the usual regimen for flare-ups.

THEME: MACROSCOPIC HAEMATURIA

13.21   F   Renal cancer

As the woman cannot see the colour of her urine she may have had haematuria for a long time. Broken bones after trivial injury raise the possibility of pathological fracture, and renal cancer typically metastasises to bone (and lungs).

CHAPTER 13 ANSWERS

13.22   J   Ureteric calculus

Stones affect more men than women and one of the classic sites where ureteric stones get lodged is the vesicoureteric junction (VUJ). Here irritation of the trigone leads to frequency and as the detrusor muscle squeezes down on itself to empty the bladder it also squeezes the stone in the VUJ leading to pain at the end of micturition.

13.23   H   Schistosomiasis

Schistosomiasis is endemic in Egypt ('the land of menstruating men,' said Herodotus) and bacterial cystitis typically coexists with the bilharzial infection, exacerbating the situation.

13.24   A   Bladder cancer

Even if the international normalised ratio (INR) is too high, bleeding usually occurs because of an abnormality somewhere along the urinary tract, and therefore patients taking warfarin need to be investigated as thoroughly as other patients. This patient is an elderly person with frank painless haematuria and therefore has approximately a 25% chance of harbouring a bladder cancer.

13.25   C   Haemorrhagic cystitis

Urinary infection is a potent cause of confusion in elderly people, and one needs to be concerned why she is not improving with the antibiotics. Either it is an unusual organism or there is a predisposing factor such as a large amount of post-void residual urine making elimination of infected urine inefficient (and contributing to long-standing urinary incontinence). Once the bladder urothelium is severely and chronically inflamed it will start to bleed.

THEME: SHORT STATURE IN CHILDREN

13.26   A   Achondroplasia

Disproportionately shortened limbs would point to a skeletal dysplasia such as achondroplasia. This is an autosomal dominant condition.

13.27   F   Noonan syndrome

Noonan syndrome in boys mimics many of the features of Turner syndrome. However, Turner occurs only in girls as it is due to the chromosomal defect XO. The mode of transmission of Noonan syndrome is thought to be autosomal dominant with variable expression.

13.28   D   Growth hormone deficiency

Cranial irradiation especially at a young age can lead to hypopituitarism and loss of growth hormone production, further resulting in short stature and hypoglycaemia.

13.29   B   Congenital hypothyroidism

The child has congenital hypothyroidism. It is detected usually by neonatal screening before the signs are evident.

THEME: CAUSES OF A NON-BLANCHING RASH

13.30   E   Henoch–Schönlein purpura

Henoch–Schönlein purpura is a hypersensitivity reaction, sometimes preceded by an upper respiratory tract infection. Associated problems include arthralgia, abdominal pain and microscopic haematuria. Glomerulonephritis can progress to renal failure so any proteinuria should be monitored. The main treatment is with analgesics. Most children recover fully over a few months.

13.31   F   Immune thrombocytopenic purpura

This is an immune disorder characterised by platelet-bound antibodies. There is often a previous history of infection. Most episodes resolve over a few months but there is a danger of serious bleeding.

13.32   H   Non-accidental injury

Always consider child abuse if purpura is seen in an unusual place or shows an unusual distribution.

13.33   G   Meningococcal septicaemia

Meningococcal purpura implies significant septicaemia. Rapid deterioration is likely. Aggressive management with antibiotics, intravenous fluids, intubation and ventilation is required.

13.34   A   Acute leukaemia

The history suggests low haemoglobin and platelets as well as poor immunity. In leukaemia all three blood cell types are affected.

THEME: INVESTIGATIONS OF PRURITUS VULVAE

13.35   C   High vaginal swab

13.36   E   None of the above

13.37   A   Creatinine clearance

13.38   D   Vulval biopsy

13.39   B   Glucose tolerance test

In most cases of pruritus vulvae there is an underlying gynaecological cause. However, in a proportion of cases systemic disorders are aetiological factors such as diabetes mellitus or dermatological conditions. Poor hygiene, use of talcum powders, deodorants, bath salts, synthetic underwear, tight jeans and biological washing powders contribute to the symptoms and these should be elicited from the history. In older women with a localised lesion, a biopsy is essential.

THEME: CAUSES OF CLUBBING

13.40   J   Infective endocarditis

Infective endocarditis is easily overlooked as a cause of subacute or chronic illness in older people. However, fever and murmurs often coexist without endocarditis. Endocarditis on a previously normal valve is more common after surgical instrumentation of the urogenital or gastro-intestinal tract or after dental work. Clinical signs include clubbing, splinter haemorrhages, haematuria, retinal Roth spots (basically cotton wool spots due to vasculitis), Janeway lesions (palmar/plantar infarcted papules) and Osler nodes (painful infarcted papules on the finger pulps).

13.41   B   Bronchiectasis

Any chronic suppurative lung disease can cause clubbing. In a young or middle-aged person, the most likely diagnosis is bronchiectasis. This may be idiopathic or follow previous infection (whooping cough, tuberculosis) or bronchial obstruction, which causes localised bronchiectasis. Signs are due to fixed narrowing of some airways with excess sputum production. In a younger patient, cystic fibrosis gives a similar clinical picture, including clubbing.

CHAPTER 13 ANSWERS

13.42   E   Squamous cell lung cancer

Smoking and asbestos exposure together massively increase the risk of lung malignancy. Squamous cell carcinoma is more common than mesothelioma and Horner syndrome is usually due to an apical squamous cell cancer.

13.43   C   Coeliac disease

Cystic fibrosis, coeliac disease and Crohn disease can all cause malabsorption, growth delay and clubbing. Of these, coeliac disease is the most common condition to present at this age. Cystic fibrosis is almost always identified in young children and most will have respiratory problems at the time of diagnosis. Children with coeliac disease are often pale skinned with fair hair. Arthralgia and dermatitis herpetiformis may also occur.

13.44   A   Axillary artery aneurysm

Unilateral clubbing is rare. One cause is an axillary artery aneurysm, which is usually acquired in adulthood after trauma such as angiography via the brachial artery. Another possibility is coarctation of the aorta proximal to the origin of the right subclavian artery.

THEME: COMMON PRESENTATIONS OF SPORTSMEN/WOMEN

13.45   J   Ulnar collateral ligament rupture

This is rupture of the ulnar collateral ligament of the thumb and is a common skiing injury. The lesion is detected on stress testing. Referral for surgical repair may be necessary, especially if the proximal end of the tendon is trapped inside the aponeurosis of the thumb adductor causing impaired abduction/adduction of the thumb. The common term is gamekeeper's thumb as it can occur when wringing a pheasant's neck!

13.46 H Shin splints

Shin splints is pain in the anterior shin caused by either a stress fracture of the tibia, inflammation of the muscles on the anterior compartment of the lower leg or periostitis of the tibia. It is an overuse syndrome caused by poor running technique where the foot is forcibly plantarflexed against resistance from tibialis anterior. The most important diagnosis to exclude is chronic compartment syndrome, where there is so much swelling that the pressure causes muscle ischaemia, more swelling and a vicious circle. In the short term, the condition can be managed by rest, and in the long term, by improving running technique with appropriate advice from an experienced physiotherapist.

13.47 D Lateral epicondylitis

Lateral epicondylitis is usually called tennis elbow but is also very common in other repeated activities involving forced pronation and extension of the wrist. Violinists present with right arm symptoms. Gripping and wrist extension are painful. The diagnosis is made by demonstrating tenderness over the lateral epicondyle, pain on resisted wrist extension. An important differential is cervical root pain, which is also common in violinists. Treatment is initially rest, ice and non-steroidal anti-inflammatory drugs (NSAIDs), followed by advice on technique, stretching and strengthening exercises from a specialist physiotherapist. Short-term relief may be obtained by local steroid injection but this does not remove the cause so there is risk of recurrence.

13.48 B Bucket handle meniscus tear

A bucket handle tear describes a common injury to the medial meniscus, caused by twisting with the knee flexed. The knee may lock or give way as the loose meniscus fragment lodges between the femoral condyles. The medial joint line will be tender and McMurray's test may be positive. There may be an effusion. Large tears may need removal of the loose body during arthroscopy; small tears may need no treatment. Refer for arthroscopy if symptoms are severe and interfere with functioning of the knee.

CHAPTER 13 ANSWERS

13.49   A   Anterior knee pain

Anterior knee pain (patellofemoral syndrome) is caused by irritation of the undersurface of the patella which may cause damage to the cartilage. The patella normally slides up and down the patellar groove on the anterior distal femur. If it is malaligned there is increased force of friction. Malalignment is usually caused by imbalance of forces between medial and lateral quadriceps groups, pulling the patella laterally. It is common in rowers because of the positioning, and in females because of the greater angle between tibia and femur caused by the wider pelvis. Initial treatment is rest, followed by exercises to strengthen the medial quadriceps and advice on technique.

THEME: HEADACHE

13.50   C   Migraine

Migraine is the most likely diagnosis. The patient is describing some classic features of migraine with some aura. The oral contraceptive should be stopped in view of this diagnosis. If simple analgesics are not beneficial then a 5HT agonist (triptan) may be helpful.

13.51   B   Cluster headache

Cluster headaches more commonly affect men and can start at any age. They are unilateral and always on the same side. They last 20–60 minutes and may recur several times every day for several weeks. Treatment is often very difficult as analgesics do not usually relieve the pain as they take too long to work. Inhalation of 100% oxygen often relieves cluster headache for some people, particularly frequent cluster headaches that occur at night.

13.52   D   Subarachnoid haemorrhage

New headaches that start very suddenly (sometimes described like a sudden blow to the head) must be taken very seriously. Any patient who describes a very severe, sudden-onset headache needs to be admitted to hospital and investigated for a subarachnoid haemorrhage.

13.53   G   Trigeminal neuralgia

This is classic trigeminal neuralgia. The majority of cases are unilateral. It occurs in the distribution of one or more divisions of the trigeminal nerve, and occurs in mid to late life. Patients often describe the pain like an electric shock, which is often precipitated by cold wind, washing the face, shaving or eating. Oral carbamazepine is usually used as first-line treatment. Occasionally surgery is needed.

13.54   F   Tension headache

The pain of tension headache is typically present all day, worse in the evening. In contrast, the pain from raised intracranial pressure tends to be present on waking and persists less during the day than a tension headache. Any stresses in the patient's life should be reduced, if possible.

13.55   E   Temporal arteritis

Temporal arteritis should be diagnosed here as he has very typical symptoms. It is important not to miss this diagnosis at it is potentially sight-threatening if left untreated. High-dose steroids need to be started as soon as the diagnosis is suspected.

CHAPTER 13 ANSWERS

THEME: FAILURE TO CONCEIVE

13.56   A   Endocervical and high vaginal swab

The history and examination findings suggest possible pelvic inflammatory disease. First-line investigation would be endocervical and high vaginal swabs to detect and treat any current genital infection. Later, a hysterosalpingogram could be indicated to look for any tubal scarring but this would not be first line.

13.57   D   Pelvic ultrasound scan

This history is suggestive of polycystic ovarian syndrome (PCOS) which a normal LH/FSH ratio does not exclude. The next investigation would therefore be a pelvic ultrasound to look for the presence of polycystic ovaries. PCOS is defined as polycystic ovaries plus one or more of: amenorrhoea/oligomenorrhoea, male pattern baldness, hirsutism, acne, raised serum testosterone and LH. Management of infertility may include weight loss and treatment with metformin and clomifene.

13.58   E   Serum LH and FSH

This woman might be perimenopausal and it is important to diagnose this before embarking on other investigations. Raised LH and FSH together with low oestradiol would suggest this.

13.59   C   Karyotype analysis

This girl has features suggestive of Turner syndrome with failure of development of any secondary sexual characteristics and primary amenorrhoea. Other clinical features of Turner syndrome are shield chest, cubitus valgus, lymphoedema, short fourth metacarpal, low-set ears and hypertension. The karyotype in Turner syndrome is 45 XO.

THEME: COLONIC DISORDERS

13.60   A   Carcinoma of the caecum

Carcinoma of the caecum often presents in an insidious way, with a microcytic anaemia, weight loss and sometimes an ache or palpable mass in the right iliac fossa. The large calibre of the caecum and liquid consistency of the stool at this point allows these tumours to grow for a long period of time. Unfortunately, some of these patients receive several courses of iron tablets before the true diagnosis is made.

13.61   G   Irritable bowel syndrome

Irritable bowel syndrome (IBS) is often a diagnosis of exclusion, which typically occurs in younger patients and may be associated with stress or dietary intolerance. Symptoms include constipation or diarrhoea or both together, along with cramp-like abdominal pains. Treatment with anti-spasmodic agents, fibre, or exclusion diets can be tried, although any organic pathology must be ruled out at first. Investigations are done if symptoms are not typical, or if symptoms of IBS develop over the age of 45 when other conditions need to be ruled out.

13.62   H   Sigmoid volvulus

Sigmoid volvulus is more common in equatorial countries where the diet is rich in fibre. However, it does occur in temperate countries and usually presents with symptoms of pain and bloating, sometimes as an emergency. A plain abdominal film may demonstrate a large double colonic loop, which is said to resemble a coffee bean.

CHAPTER 13 ANSWERS

13.63   B   Carcinoma of the sigmoid colon

Left-sided colonic tumours will more commonly present with an obstructive picture than right-sided tumours. This is due to the more narrow calibre of the colon combined with the more solid consistency of its contents at this point. Typically an annular constricting carcinoma will present with an alteration in bowel habit, change in stool calibre, and finally, frank obstruction. A plain abdominal film may show gross faecal loading proximal to this point, with an absence of bowel gas distally. A contrast enema will usually confirm the diagnosis.

13.64   I   Ulcerative colitis

Ulcerative colitis is a disease of unknown aetiology which tends to affect people in the third and fourth decade of life (15% are under the age of 15). It usually presents as a chronic relatively low-grade illness, although 15% of patients may present with fulminant disease. Symptoms include blood-stained diarrhoea, abdominal pain and fever. Extracolonic manifestations include arthritis, iritis, hepatic dysfunction and cutaneous manifestations. The ulceration is superficial, unlike the transmural disease seen in Crohn colitis.

THEME: MONITORING OF DRUGS

13.65   E   Phenytoin

The relationship between dose and plasma concentration is not linear. Small dose increases may produce large increases in plasma concentrations with a risk of toxic effects.

13.66   B   Azathioprine

There is a risk of bone marrow depression.

13.67   D   Lithium

Lithium salts have a narrow therapeutic/toxic ratio. Doses are adjusted to achieve a serum concentration of 0.4–1.0mmol/l on samples taken 12 hours after a dose. Lithium also causes hypothyroidism.

13.68   F   Ramipril

Angiotensin-converting enzyme (ACE) inhibitors are likely to cause progressive renal failure in patients with renal artery stenosis and in certain other situations.

THEME: CAUSES OF A SORE MOUTH

13.69   D   Geographic tongue

Geographic tongue or erythema migrans is a common autosomal dominant inherited condition that may affect up to 5% of the population. The dorsum of the tongue is affected with migratory areas of depapillation, which may be surrounded by whitish margins. It is often asymptomatic but can give rise to concern when first noticed by the patient or if it leads to soreness while eating spicy food.

13.70   H   Squamous cell carcinoma

Oral squamous cell carcinoma is the commonest oral malignancy. Its preferred site is the U-shaped area in the floor of the mouth that lies between and includes the lateral border of the tongue and the mucosa covering the lingual aspect of mandibular alveolar bone. Note that a biopsy should be done for any oral ulcer which has persisted for more than 2 weeks to exclude malignancy. White and red patches in the mouth may be dysplastic or represent carcinoma.

CHAPTER 13 ANSWERS

13.71   F   Lichen planus

Lichen planus is a mucocutaneous disorder of possibly immunological aetiology. The eruption both on the skin and in the mouth tends to be symmetrical. On the skin it tends to start on the flexor surfaces with red and then violaceous pruritic, polygonal, papules, which may have white 'Wickham' striae on their surface. In about 50% of patients the skin lesions resolve within 9 months. Oral lesions tend to continue for much longer and may be reticular, atrophic or ulcerative. The genitalia may also be involved. Lichen planus, like psoriasis, viral warts and vitiligo, shows the Koebner phenomenon (lesions spread into traumatised areas, eg along a scratch mark).

13.72   E   Iron deficiency

Iron deficiency may present initially with angular cheilitis and a smooth, red, depapillated, sore tongue. The cause of iron deficiency in this patient may be an occult caecal carcinoma.

13.73   J   Thrush

Poor steroid inhaler technique often results in patients with asthma developing steroid-associated oral candidosis or thrush which may cause an erythematous appearance of the dorsum of the tongue and opposing palate. All patients starting to use such inhalers should have their technique checked, should rinse their mouth after inhaler use and if possible use a spacer device to increase delivery of the corticosteroid to the lungs.

THEME: CHILD WITH A PAINFUL LEG

13.74   F   Perthes disease

Perthes disease generally presents with limp, with or without pain, between the ages of 4 and 8 years. Avascular necrosis of the femoral head occurs followed by replacement with new bone. The patient can be left with residual femoral head deformity. Other causes of avascular necrosis in children are sickle cell disease and prolonged steroid use. It is unlikely to be sickle cell disease as this would be associated with severe pain and there would have been a history of other crises by the age of 5 years.

13.75   J   Slipped femoral epiphysis

Slipped upper femoral epiphysis can present with pain and a limp of gradual onset, or more acutely after minor trauma. It presents at this age and classically in obese boys with delayed secondary sexual development.

13.76   D   Osgood–Schlatter disease

This is a traction apophysitis at the insertion of the patellar tendon into the tibial tubercle. Tenderness over the tubercle and changes seen on X-ray confirm the diagnosis. Treatment involves reducing the strain at this site by stopping sports or by immobilisation.

13.77   B   Irritable hip

In this age group the joint may become inflamed after an upper respiratory tract infection. The exact cause is not known but it causes an irritable hip or transient synovitis. Blood tests and X-rays show normal findings. Most cases resolve in a few days or weeks. This diagnosis is made only once all investigations are demonstrated to be normal.

CHAPTER 13 ANSWERS

13.78   C   Non-accidental injury

The pathological diagnosis is likely to be fractured femur. However, the clinical diagnosis may be non-accidental injury. Infants are unlikely to break their bones without some external force. Children might be brought in by carers other than the parents. A senior paediatric opinion must be sought immediately while you attend to the child's injury.

13.79   C   Toxic shock syndrome

Toxic shock syndrome usually occurs in the setting of staphylococcal infection of skin or soft tissues, and is mediated by the endotoxin TSS-1. Characteristic clinical features also include hypotension, shock and very high body temperatures (> 39.5°C). Treatment is predominantly with supportive care to ensure adequate circulating volume, administration of pressor agents to maintain systemic blood pressure and antibiotic treatment. The first thing to do is to remove the tampon, which is the likely source of the infection in this case.

13.80   A   Fasting blood sugar

Granuloma annulare is slightly more common in women. It is associated with type 1 diabetes, which if present can be diagnosed by fasting glucose. HbA1c is not sensitive enough to test for diabetes and is usually used to monitor ongoing control. Granuloma annulare itself is harmless and self-limiting.

13.81   C   Parvovirus infection

Parvovirus causes erythema infectiosum (Fifth disease) characterised by a prodromal illness with fever followed by an erythematous facial rash (slapped cheek appearance).

The following diseases are notifiable: acute encephalitis; acute poliomyelitis; anthrax; cholera; diphtheria; dysentery; food poisoning; leptospirosis; malaria; measles; meningitis (meningococcal, pneumococcal, *Haemophilus influenzae*, viral, other specified, unspecified*)*; meningococcal septicaemia (without meningitis); mumps; ophthalmia neonatorum; paratyphoid fever; plague; rabies; relapsing fever; rubella; scarlet fever; smallpox; tetanus; tuberculosis; typhoid fever; typhus fever; viral haemorrhagic fever; viral hepatitis (hepatitis A, hepatitis B, hepatitis C, other); whooping cough; yellow fever; and leprosy.

13.82   B   Autoimmune hepatitis

There are two peaks according to age in the presentation. Patients in the perimenopausal age group present with non-specific symptoms, whereas adolescents and people in their early twenties present with acute hepatitis and with jaundice and higher aminotransferase levels, which do not improve with time. Three types of autoimmune hepatitis have been recognised:

- type I with antibodies (antinuclear anti-smooth muscle)
- type II with antibodies (anti-LKM1)
- type III with soluble liver antigen.

Type II mostly occurs in girls and young women.

CHAPTER 13 ANSWERS

13.83   D   Tachypnoea > 25 breaths/minute

PEFR in an acute severe attack is less than 33% predicted, and tachycardia is greater than 120 beats/minute. Other signs of life-threatening asthma include use of accessory muscles of respiration, inability to complete sentences in one breath, confusion or exhaustion and a silent chest. Acute attacks may build up over minutes, hours or days, and there may be a wide range of precipitants. These include smoking, infection, stress, allergens, exercise and neglect of medications.

13.84   A   Brisk biceps reflex

Brisk reflexes are an upper motor neurone sign and suggest spinal cord compression above the level of lesion. There may be lower motor neurone signs at the level of the lesion. The level of biceps reflex is C5–6. The other signs are all common in self-limiting cervicalgia.

13.85   B   A 24-year-old unemployed single man

Although all of the above people do have an increased risk of attempting suicide, the risk is greatest in the young man. Single, unemployed men from the lower social classes have a high risk of suicide, and any voiced intention must be taken very seriously in the consultation.

13.86   D   Hypothyroidism

All the other options are established risk factors for stroke. Primary prevention of stroke is very important in primary care. Also much of the responsibility for delivering effective secondary prevention and managing longer-term problems associated with stroke now falls to the primary care team.

13.87 E Secondary post-partum haemorrhage

The difference between primary and secondary post-partum haemorrhage (PPH) is the timing of bleeding after delivery. Primary PPH usually occurs 24–48 hours after delivery, whereas secondary PPH can occur from 48 hours up to 14 days after delivery. In this clinical scenario, secondary PPH is due to endometritis (an infection caused by bacterial penetration of the residual stratum basalis of the endometrium), as suggested by the raised temperature, offensive vaginal discharge and tender uterus. The underlying aggravating factor may be retained products of conception, which provide a rich culture medium for the growth of bacteria.

13.88 D The dose of the drug is 500mg twice daily

Lesser doses are likely to be ineffective. Improvement is slow with only about 20% improvement after 1 month. If the drug is effective it is usual to continue for 6 months or longer. Inflamed lesions usually respond better to oral antibiotics and it is usual to also prescribe a topical retinoid if there are a significant number of comedones. Oxytetracycline reduces the efficacy of the combined oral contraceptive by impairing the bacterial flora responsible for recycling ethinyloestradiol from the large bowel. The British National Formulary states that if the course of treatment exceeds 3 weeks, the bacterial flora develop anti-bacterial resistance and additional precautions become unnecessary unless a new antibacterial is prescribed.[4]

13.89 C Phenytoin

Gingival overgrowth, also known as gingival hyperplasia secondary to drugs, was first reported in the literature in the early 1960s in institutionalised epileptic children receiving phenytoin for the treatment of seizures. Ciclosporin and calcium channel blockers (especially nifedipine) have also been associated with gingival overgrowth. In patients taking phenytoin it is more likely to occur in the presence of gingivitis and dental plaque. Increased dental plaque induces local inflammation and may serve as a reservoir for the drug.

CHAPTER 13 ANSWERS

13.90   B   Patients with a 10-year cardiovascular disease risk of more than 20% should receive a statin for primary prevention

Statins are now widely prescribed for both primary and secondary prevention of coronary heart disease.[5] All type 2 diabetic patients should be receiving a statin for primary prevention of cardiovascular disease (unless contraindicated). Fibrates are used first line to lower very high triglyceride levels. Only hypertensive patients with a 10-year risk of more than 20% should be considered for a statin.

13.91   B   Fasting glucose 8.1mmol/l

The World Health Organization's publication *Definition, Diagnosis and Classification of Diabetes Mellitus and its Complications* (1999)[6] defines the diagnostic criteria as follows:

Diabetes symptoms (ie polyuria, polydipsia and unexplained weight loss) plus

- a random venous plasma glucose concentration ≥ 11.1mmol/l

or

- a fasting plasma glucose concentration ≥ 7.0mmol/l (whole blood ≥ 6.1mmol/l)

or

- 2-hour plasma glucose concentration ≥ 11.1mmol/l 2 hours after 75g anhydrous glucose in an oral glucose tolerance test (OGTT).

When there are no symptoms, diagnosis should not be based on a single glucose determination and requires confirmatory plasma venous determination. At least one additional glucose test result on another day with a value in the diabetic range is essential: fasting, from a random sample or from the 2-hour post glucose load. If the fasting or random values are not diagnostic the 2-hour value should be used. HbA1c should never be used to diagnose diabetes.

13.92   A   A 12-hour-old baby with jaundice

Jaundice that appears in less than 24 hours may be pathological and needs to be investigated. All other answers are normal variants in babies. The rash described in F refers to Epstein's pearls and in B refers to erythema toxicum (neonatal urticaria), which are both normal. A newborn baby commonly sneezes to remove amniotic fluid from the nose. Blue hands and feet are common in the first few days of life in a baby. Post-dates babies often have very dry skin.

13.93   A   *Borrelia burgdorferi* infection

Borrelia causes Lyme disease, treated with doxycycline or erythromycin. Strictly speaking it is a spirochaete, but the deer tick which transmits it is a parasite. In the UK it is endemic in Thetford Forest (Norfolk), the New Forest, the Lake District, the Scottish Highlands and the uplands of Wales. Twenty per cent of patients with Lyme disease do not remember any tick bites and do not complain of a rash. If the tick bites at the nymph stage it is often not felt because of local anaesthetic secretions. The initial rash known as erythema chronicum migrans is a macule or papule at the bite site that expands to form an annular lesion with a distinct red border and a partially clearing centre.

13.94   E   Treat with broad-spectrum antibiotics

This scenario describes a patient with diverticulitis. Features on history are the lower abdominal pain/LIF pain with nausea and constipation. The patient may look flushed. It is more common with age, and in females. A low fibre diet is a risk factor. As this woman is able to tolerate fluids and you do not suspect any complications such as obstruction or abscess, then appropriate management is with broad-spectrum antibiotics, such as ciprofloxacin and metronidazole for 1 week and a clear liquid diet.

CHAPTER 13 ANSWERS

13.95   B   ESR

Polymyalgia rheumatica is characterised by raised ESR and C-reactive protein (CRP) levels. The diagnosis should be questioned if these levels are not raised. Serum alkaline phosphatase and γ-glutamyl transferase may also be elevated. A temporal artery biopsy shows giant-cell arteritis in about 10–30% of cases, but is usually not done.

13.96   B   Add insulin glargine

Insulin glargine has reduced solubility due to its modified structure, thus prolonging its duration of action. Therefore it has a less peaked concentration profile in the blood than conventional long-acting insulins. It is recommended that it should be available for those whose lifestyle is considerably restricted by recurrent symptomatic hypoglycaemia.[7]

13.97   A   Alzheimer disease

People particularly at risk of developing Alzheimer disease are those with a family history of the disease, those who have sustained a head injury or those who have Down syndrome. Neuropathological changes include neuronal reduction, neurofibrillary tangles, senile neurotic plaques and a variable amyloid angiopathy. Aggregation of amyloid appears to be a central event. The gene for the amyloid precursor protein (APP) is localised close to the defect on chromosome 21. Dementia is diagnosed clinically from the patient's history and examination, especially cognitive testing, and it can be confirmed by psychometric testing.

13.98   B   Check for serum varicella zoster IgG

If a susceptible mother is exposed to a source of varicella zoster virus, then this may result in primary varicella infection in pregnancy. Maternal varicella in the first 20 weeks of pregnancy carries a 1–2% risk of varicella embryopathy syndrome developing in the fetus. The consequences of fetal varicella syndrome include scarring of the skin, hypoplasia of limbs and chorioretinitis. Adult varicella can cause pneumonitis as a serious complication. In the absence of symptoms, positive IgG antibody levels are highly suggestive of past infection and hence immunity.

13.99   E   Peyronie disease

Peyronie disease presents with hard lumps in the shaft of the penis and pain and bending on erection. The cause is unknown. Although it can cause erectile dysfunction, it does not affect fertility or sperm count. All of the other answers are well recognised causes of reduced fertility in men.

13.100   B   Acute otitis media

The history is short so this is an acute condition. In otitis externa the pain would not improve when the ear discharges. In otitis media a rupture of the tympanic membrane releasing discharge reduces the pain. Glue ear and wax usually just produce deafness.

CHAPTER 13 ANSWERS

REFERENCES

1. National Institute for Health and Clinical Excellence. *Hypertension: Management of hypertension in adults in primary care* (homepage on the Internet), June 2006 (cited 2008 May 10). Available from http://www.nice.org.uk/CG034

2. Wiysonge CS, Bradley H, Mayosi BM, Maroney R, Mbewu A, Opie LH, Volmink J. *Beta-blockers for hypertension*. Cochrane Database of Systematic Reviews 2007, Issue 1. Art. No.: CD002003. DOI: 10.1002/14651858.CD002003.pub2.

3. *Drugs acting on the oropharynx*. 12.3. British National Formulary; 55; 2008.

4. *Combined hormonal contraceptives*. 7.3.1. British National Formulary; 55; 2008.

5. British Cardiac Society, British Hypertension Society, Diabetes UK, HEART UK, Primary Care Cardiovascular Society, The Stroke Association; *JBS 2: Joint British Societies' guidelines on prevention of cardiovascular disease in clinical practice*. Heart 2005; 91;1-52.

6. *Definition, Diagnosis and Classification of Diabetes Mellitus and its Complications*. Report of a WHO Consultation. Geneva: World Health Organization 1999.

7. *Intermediate and long acting insulins*. 6.1.1.2. British National Formulary; 55; 2008.

Professional
Dilemmas

INTRODUCTION TO PROFESSIONAL DILEMMA QUESTIONS

Professional dilemma questions make up the second paper in the Stage 2 assessment process of appointment to general practitioner (GP) specialty training. Candidates have 105 minutes to complete this paper. The paper focuses on a candidate's approach to practising medicine. It consists of scenarios of professional dilemmas that might be met when practising as a doctor. Candidates have to decide how to deal with them. Thus the paper is designed to assess understanding of appropriate behaviour for a doctor in difficult situations and allows the demonstration of competencies such as coping with pressure, empathy and sensitivity, and professional integrity. These are three of the competencies in the national person specification for entry at ST1 level into GP training.[1]

The paper does not require any specific knowledge of general practice but does assume a general familiarity with typical primary and secondary care procedures. A candidate's responses should represent appropriate behaviour for a second year foundation doctor.

The competencies that are assessed are:

- Empathy and sensitivity: This is the capacity and motivation to take into account others' perspectives and understand their concerns but without over-sensitive involvement. The patient will be treated with understanding using a non-judgemental approach and with appropriate words and actions.

- Coping with pressure: This is the ability to recognise one's own limitations and to seek help where necessary. It requires coping mechanisms to remain under control of difficult situations, maintain the wider focus and respond appropriately when faced with the unexpected.

- Professional integrity: This means having the capacity and motivation to take responsibility and accept challenges, to admit and learn from mistakes and to demonstrate respect and equality of care for all. Patients' needs will be put before one's own when appropriate.

On the following pages are examples of typical questions in these three areas. The examples also demonstrate the two main question formats:

- Where rank ordering is required a correct order has been decided by consensus of a panel of general practitioners. Full marks will be obtained when the choices are put in the correct order. A small variation such as reversing the first and second options will only result in a small reduction in marks. A zero mark is only given when the whole order is reversed by a candidate.

- Where a candidate has to choose possible correct options from a list then a mark is awarded for each correct item chosen.

Example 1

Question You are a foundation doctor working on a busy surgical unit. On theatre days you often find you have to deal with difficult ward problems without adequate supervision from senior colleagues. You are unhappy about this.

Rank the possible responses below in the most suitable order.

1 Discuss the situation with your consultant

2 Discuss the situation with your foundation programme director

3 Seek advice from experienced nurses on the unit when in difficulty

4 Seek advice from other foundation colleagues when you have difficulty

Answer 1 2 4 3

This question deals with coping with pressure and, in particular, recognising limitations and establishing effective strategies. Foundation doctors should always have easy access to senior cover. The person most likely to be able to sort things out is your consultant and failing that your programme director who should have influence over the way foundation doctors are trained in the hospital. Both the other options are inappropriate but asking doctors is slightly better than asking nurses because of the nature of their training.

Example 2

Question You are in a general practice surgery. A 40-year-old man whom you referred to hospital with abdominal pain was found to have multiple liver and peritoneal metastases from an earlier colonic carcinoma. The local oncologist thinks he is unsuitable for chemotherapy and is now terminally ill. He has been advised by a family member who is a nurse at a regional oncology centre to see a specialist there who does clinical trials and he asks if you can refer him.

Rank the possible responses below in the most suitable order.

1 Advise him that this is not a suitable option

2 Discuss with him his feelings and expectations about a possible referral

3 Speak to the local oncologist about the request

4 Speak to the regional specialist about the request

Answer 2 3 4 1

This question deals with empathy and sensitivity and in particular responding to the needs and concerns of the patient. None of these options are wrong and indeed it is unlikely that chemotherapy will help him. However, the main issue here is to find out what the patient is thinking and what he feels his needs are. As he has asked for a referral this is most likely what he wants. Professional etiquette dictates that you talk to the local oncologist first. He may be able to advise you and perhaps even make the referral himself.

Example 3

Question You are in a general practice surgery. A 50-year-old man has a red scaly lesion behind one ear. Two years earlier a local dermatologist was quite definite about a diagnosis of seborrhoeic eczema and he prescribed a moderately potent steroid cream. The patient does not think the cream was effective when he used it 2 years ago. He has had no treatment since and has come back to see you in the GP surgery because the lesion is still present. There is a small area of ulceration in the centre and you are concerned he may be developing a squamous cell carcinoma.

Select from the list below the three most suitable responses at this consultation.

1 Arrange a biopsy to be carried out in the practice

2 Ask your supervisor to come in and have a look at the lesion

3 Offer to review him in 1 month to see if there is any worsening of the lesion

4 Prescribe a more potent steroid

5 Prescribe the same steroid that he had 2 years ago

6 Refer him back to the original consultant

7 Refer him to a different consultant

Answer 1 2 6

This question is in the area of professional integrity and in particular a willingness to back one's own professional judgement. Here you are told that you suspect the lesion is a squamous cell carcinoma. This means that you think the consultant made an incorrect diagnosis and presumably the diagnosis should have been that of a precancerous lesion such as actinic keratosis or Bowen disease. It is hard for a junior doctor to contradict a senior colleague. If there is an easily available second opinion such as the clinical supervisor then it is obvious that this should be the first course of action. If you are correct then the patient needs an urgent biopsy either in hospital or the practice. The original consultant should have the opportunity to know about and learn from his mistake and a referral to another consultant would only be appropriate if the patient expressed a preference for this. None of the other options are appropriate.

The personal skills that are being tested in Stage 2 should have been acquired during undergraduate and foundation training so no special preparation should be necessary apart from becoming familiar with the format of the test. It is useful to discuss a variety of issues with educational supervisors. In particular, discuss the wider issues involved in the complex medical and management problems encountered in everyday practice. Also, regular case analysis and discussion with colleagues is a good way to practise and develop competences in this area.

The necessary attributes of a doctor are defined by the General Medical Council and can be accessed via their website[2] or through their various publications, particularly *Good Medical Practice*.[3]

REFERENCES

1. The National Recruitment Office for General Practice Training website (http://www.gprecruitment.org.uk).

2 General Medical Council. *Good Medical Practice* (2006). Available at: http://www.gmc-uk.org/guidance/good_medical_practice

3. General Medical Council. *Good Medical Practice*. London: General Medical Council, 2006.

Chapter 14
Professional
Dilemmas

QUESTIONS

14.1 You are a foundation doctor in the Emergency Department. A 40-year-old man complains of a flu-like illness for 1 week with cough but no shortness of breath. He is apyrexial and has a clear chest. The patient informs you that he is a consultant anaesthetist from Australia on holiday in the UK. He demands antibiotics, specifically an expensive new one which is rarely used in the UK but 'we use it all the time back home for chest infections'.

Rank the possible responses below in the most suitable order.

1 Advise him that it is good practice not to prescribe antibiotics immediately for a flu-like illness, that he should take symptomatic relief and consult a doctor again if things get worse or do not improve in a reasonable amount of time

2 Ask for advice from your consultant/registrar on the shop floor

3 Politely ask him if he can give evidence of his professional qualifications before prescribing

4 Respect his expectation and prescribe the requested antibiotic

14.2 You are a foundation doctor in psychiatry. You cover a busy acute psychiatric ward, divided into two groups, each under a different consultant. You gradually realise that the other trainee cannot cope with her work. She frequently hides in the doctor's office, does not complete the tasks requested by the nurses, and rarely reviews her patients by herself. However, she takes good notes from ward rounds and her consultant does not seem to have any issues with her work. No-one else has yet commented on this. You can only just manage the workload from the patients under your consultant.

Rank the possible responses below in the most suitable order.

1 Cover your colleague's work

2 Discuss the problem with her consultant

3 Report her to hospital management

4 Raise the issue directly with your colleague

14.3 Nursing staff tell you the 19-year-old son of one of your patients is waiting to talk with you about his mother's condition. She has just been told she has breast cancer and is about to undergo further investigations to determine the management.

Rank the possible responses below in the most suitable order.

1 Offer to discuss things with his mother present

2 Read the patient's notes, and take them in with you to fully provide any information the son needs about his mother

3 See the son, listen to his concerns and explain about any procedures he is worried about without revealing any confidential information

4 Tell the nursing staff to tell the son to discuss it with his mother

14.4 You are a foundation doctor based in a busy GP surgery for 4 months. Unfortunately all the consulting rooms are occupied and you can only see patients in surgery between the hours of 11:30 and 14:00.

Rank the possible responses below in the most suitable order.

1   Discuss with the practice manager to try to identify possible slots in which you can reschedule some of your surgeries

2   Feel that it is better not to complain and accept the situation

3   Report the practice to the foundation programme director

4   Use the rest of the time to sit in with other team members or seek alternative activities in the practice

14.5   **During the final week of your foundation attachment in general practice a patient you have been looking after gives you a thank you card. Inside, you find a cheque for £200.**

Rank the possible responses below in the most suitable order.

1   Happily accept the gift as a just reward for your efforts

2   Identify your feeling of embarrassment at receiving the gift and refuse

3   Offer to use the money to buy some equipment for the surgery

4   Politely talk to the patient to ascertain the reason for the gift

14.6   **You suspect that a colleague in your hospital firm is misusing alcohol. He seems sober when at work but at mess parties and when out socially you have noticed that he usually gets quite drunk.**

Rank the possible responses below in the most suitable order.

1   Discuss matters with him directly as you know him well

2   Discuss matters with other colleagues to get their views

3   Discuss matters with your consultant or the firm's clinical director

4   Report him to the General Medical Council (GMC)

14.7   You are working in the Emergency Department. A 30-year-old woman complains of shortness of breath, chest pain and shaking hands. She does not smoke and has no family history of note. She also complains of tingling around her mouth. Her observations are normal blood pressure, pulse of 100 and respiratory rate of 15–18 (variable). An electrocardiogram (ECG) is normal, and examination is normal apart from these observations. She is very anxious. You diagnose a panic attack and reassure her that the problem is not heart or lung related, and discharge her. After she is gone your registrar, who had not seen the patient, reviews the case and says that with a tachycardia and shortness of breath we should exclude a pulmonary embolism and she should have had a D-dimer test. He recommends you call her back in for this.

Rank the possible responses below in the most suitable order.

1   Arrange for the patient to be called back immediately for the test

2   Discuss with the registrar that your clinical judgement was that she did not have a serious physical illness and that you did take a proper history and examine her

3   Learn from this and consider doing more investigations in future before discharging a patient

4   Telephone the patient, see how she is feeling, and depending on the outcome you may offer investigations

14.8 You are a foundation doctor on rotation in general practice. During a consultation, a patient complains about the attitude of one of the reception staff. What do you do?

Rank the possible responses below in the most suitable order.

1 Address the complaint with the member of staff directly

2 Outline the practice's complaints procedure and ask the patient to speak to the practice manager

3 Try to calm the patient's concerns and stop this complaint becoming more serious

4 Raise the incident at the next partners' meeting (meeting between doctors in the practice)

14.9 In your work as a foundation doctor in general practice you find one of the receptionists having a look at the medical records of a patient you have seen that morning. The patient and her family are well known to the practice as frequent consulters and live in the house next door.

Rank the possible responses below in the most suitable order.

1 Address your concerns about records at the practice meeting

2 Discuss the matter with your trainer

3 Informally ask the receptionist what she is doing

4 Report the matter to the practice manager

14.10 You are in general practice visiting an 86-year-old man with moderately severe chronic obstructive pulmonary disease, complaining of worsening shortness of breath. He frequently calls out general practitioners and is occasionally admitted to hospital for a few days. The respiratory nurse specialists visit him fortnightly to avoid unnecessary admissions, and had sent a note to the practice the previous day saying that he was very anxious but they did not consider admission necessary. On examination his pulse is 100 and regular and he is tachypnoeic. His oxygen saturation is 94% on air, which is normal for him. On auscultating his chest, there are widespread coarse crackles. He says that he will not cope at home tonight and begs to be admitted to hospital. He admits to being lonely and prefers the hospital as he receives more attention.

Rank the possible responses below in the most suitable order.

1 Admit him to hospital

2 Advise him that he is no worse than usual and that you will not admit him

3 Discuss with the patient benefits of admission versus staying at home

4 Telephone the hospital 'rapid response' admission avoidance team

14.11 You are in general practice and your surgery is running half an hour late. Your patient is a 35-year-old woman with chronic back pain and sciatica who takes regular paracetamol, tramadol and gabapentin. She also has moderate depression with occasional severe exacerbations and takes citalopram. She has a history of repeated deliberate self-harm. The patient asks for a repeat prescription of all her pain medications, as the last supply issued 1 week ago has gone missing from her flat. You notice before she comes in that in the previous consultation last week she was referred to the acute mental health home treatment team because of suicidal thoughts following a recent relationship breakdown. When you mention this, she assures you that she no longer feels suicidal and is taking her citalopram regularly. She says it is mainly the pain that is getting her down.

Rank the possible responses below in the most suitable order.

1 Ask her to wait in the waiting room and phone the home treatment team and ask for their opinion on her mental state and suicide risk, and find out their plans

2 Examine her mental state further before prescribing

3 Issue her with a week's supply of medication

4 Issue the prescription and plan to telephone the home treatment team after surgery

14.12 **As a foundation doctor in general practice you notice some old and new bruises on the legs of a woman who you often see with minor illnesses. You suspect domestic violence. What do you do?**

Rank the possible responses below in the most suitable order.

1 Call social services and ask for a domestic assessment

2 Contact her partner, also a patient of yours, and ask him what he has been doing to her

3 Ignore the bruises and hope that she will ask for help when she feels ready

4 Raise the issue by asking her how she sustained the bruises

14.13 It is the weekend and the plastic surgery ward staff asks you to prescribe analgesia for one of their postoperative patients. When you go to see the patient it is clear he/she finds you attractive, and he/she tells you they have just ended a long-term relationship and are looking for a fresh start. The patient says that he/she will be discharged the following day, and asks you out on a date the following weekend.

Rank the possible responses below in the most suitable order.

1 Discuss the matter with colleagues

2 Gently explain that your duties of a doctor preclude any relationship

3 Report him/her to the hospital management for sexual harassment

4 Wait until he/she is discharged before accepting

14.14 You are a foundation doctor coming to the end of a busy surgical job, and your colleague working on the same ward contracts chickenpox. He may be absent for up to 4 weeks. You usually cover the ward for each other to attend clinic twice per week and to assist in theatre whenever possible. You do not think you will be able to cope with all the work alone.

Rank the possible responses below in the most suitable order.

1 Arrange cover with other colleagues

2 Complain to hospital management of overwork

3 Discuss your workload with your consultant

4 Make sure outpatients is informed that you may be called away

14.15 You are a foundation doctor in general surgery. Your child's nursery (on the hospital site) telephones to say that your 1-year-old has a temperature of 38°C and needs to be picked up as soon as possible. Your partner is 50 miles away on business and you are due to assist your consultant in theatre.

Rank the possible responses below in the most suitable order.

1 Apologise to your consultant and go to pick up your daughter. He can arrange another assistant

2 Arrange for a colleague to cover in return for you helping them out later

3 Explain your situation to the nursery. You pay them to look after your child so they can keep her until the end of the day

4 Phone around friends to find someone else to pick up your daughter

14.16 You are working in a busy city practice. You realise that the next patient on your list is a teacher at your son's primary school. She obviously does not know it is you she is due to see. The appointment screen says the problem is 'personal'.

Rank the possible responses below in the most suitable order.

1 Arrange for another doctor to see the patient, explaining why to both him and the patient

2 Ask the patient whether she would still like to see you, or another doctor

3 See the patient, reassuring her very carefully that you are impeccably confidential

4 Make sure that everyone you know is aware of where you work to avoid this happening

14.17 You are working in the Emergency Department and see a 35-year-old lady with chest pain. You take a history from her whilst her husband and daughter are present. They leave the cubicle and whilst they are away the lady tells you that she contracted HIV a year ago whilst working as a health care assistant. She tells you that her family are not aware that she is HIV positive. What should you do?

Rank the possible responses below in the most suitable order.

1 Explore her ideas and concerns and find out why she has not told her family that she is HIV positive

2 Ignore it

3 Offer to discuss it with her husband whilst she is present

4 Strongly advise her that she should tell her husband

14.18 You are a foundation year 2 doctor working in the Emergency Department. You see a 23-year-old insulin dependent diabetic lady who has come in with 2-day history of abdominal pain and vomiting. She thinks she has got food poisoning and just wants some medications for her sickness. Blood and urine results show that she is in diabetic ketoacidosis (DKA). You need to admit her and treat the condition but she does not want to stay in hospital as she needs to pick up her son from school and has no one to look after him. What do you do?

Rank the possible responses below in the most suitable order.

1 Allow the patient to go home and pick up her son

2 Explain the severity of her condition and that it can be life threatening if not treated as quickly as possible

3 Phone a neighbour/relative who would be able look after the child

4 Phone social services

14.19 **One of the patients under your care as a foundation year 2 doctor remains unconscious following a stroke. A colleague, who practises acupuncture, says she would like to see whether this is helpful in helping the patient regain consciousness. What do you do?**

Rank the possible responses below in the most suitable order.

1 Discuss the idea with the your senior colleagues and consultant

2 Dismiss this notion as ridiculous

3 Involve the patient's family in any decision making

4 Seek advice from the hospital authorities

5 Seek advice from your defence organisation

14.20 **You are a foundation year 2 doctor working on a busy surgical firm. During the first 2 months your registrar has repeatedly shouted at you and on occasions has humiliated you in front of patients and their relatives. What actions should you take?**

Rank the possible responses below in the most suitable order.

1 Discuss the matter with your consultant

2 Do nothing; you are now halfway through the rotation and can put up with it until you finish

3 Seek advice from the BMA

4 Seek advice from the nurses on the ward

5 Talk to the registrar and find out why he is treating you in this way

14.21 You are a foundation year 2 trainee working in the Emergency Department. During one of your regular training sessions with the other junior doctors the consultant highlights the missed fractures that have been detected via routine radiology review. You recognise that one of these is a patient you saw and realise you are one of the doctors who missed a fracture. What should you do?

Choose the three most appropriate options from the list below.

1 Amend the patient's notes highlighting why this was a difficult X-ray to interpret

2 Ask for senior review of X-rays before discharging patients

3 Listen carefully to the training to see if there is anything that can improve your skills

4 Speak to the consultant to see if there are any specific learning points to be aware of

5 Stop reviewing X-rays

6 Write to the patient apologising for the mistake

14.22   You are a doctor in the Emergency Department. A colleague
on the same rota has just been accepted on to a course he
really wants to attend and asks you to cover his night shift
next Wednesday. You will be working 08:00 to 18:00 all
week and this means you would not have enough time to
get home between shifts. He offers to pay you the standard
locum rate. You will be working together for the next few
months and you do not want to offend him.

Choose the three most appropriate options from the list
below.

1   Advise your colleague to discuss the issue with his consultant and
offer to rearrange your sessions to help if needed

2   Do the night shift but call in sick the next day as it will be easier to
find locum cover in the daytime

3   Do the shift plus your own work and rely on short naps during quiet
periods to combat fatigue

4   Discuss the problem with other colleagues to formulate a solution

5   Discuss with your consultant and offer to work the night shift if the
day shifts can be covered to allow you enough rest

6   Refuse to cover him because he should have been more organised
with his study leave request

14.23   You are in general practice doing telephone triage. You speak to a patient who seems anxious and says she is 'very unwell'. She has severe sleep problems due to restless legs syndrome secondary to chronic renal failure and is due a follow up appointment at the local sleep clinic in 6 weeks' time. She has previously asked one of the partners to fax the clinic and bring the appointment forward as she is not sleeping at all. There is no mention of this in your colleague's notes, just discussion of her other medical problems. She has discontinued the medication recommended by the clinic as it was 'no use'. She becomes verbally aggressive when you try to take a more detailed history and demands you promise to send the fax straightaway.

Choose the three most appropriate options from the list below.

1   Ask her if she would mind being more polite over the telephone. Agree to write to the clinic requesting they see her sooner

2   Assure the patient you do have her interests to heart and will fax the sleep clinic straightaway

3   Discuss her anxiety and offer a further appointment in the surgery to think further about other options while waiting for the clinic appointment

4   Discuss her expectations of referral times to a non-emergency clinic and advise her to reconsider in the meantime trying the medication they recommend

5   Say you will wait until tomorrow and discuss the issue with your colleague who is not in surgery today

6   Suggest that this is not an emergency and the sleep clinic is following her up at an appropriate interval

14.24 You are working in general practice and discover an abnormal smear result (severe dyskaryosis), which has not been acted on. The result was sent to your practice 6 months ago. The practice nurse tells you that this has happened before. What steps would you take next?

Choose the three most appropriate options from the list below.

1 Ask the nurse to do a further smear today

2 Contact your medical defence society for advice

3 Discuss the issue at a practice significant event meeting

4 Send an urgent referral for colposcopy

5 Telephone the patient to come in and discuss the matter

6 Write to the patient outlining what has happened and inviting her to come and discuss the matter if she wishes

14.25 You are a foundation year 2 doctor working in the Emergency Department. You see a 5-month-old baby who has been brought in by mum; she is concerned, as she has seen blood coming out of one ear. You examine the child and note a perforated eardrum. There is poor rapport between mum and baby and you suspect non-accidental injury (NAI).

What further action should you take? Choose the three most appropriate options from the list below.

1 Discuss with the nurse in charge and ask him/her what you should do

2 Discuss the case with the paediatric consultant

3 Find out if the child is already on the child protection register

4 Report the incident to social services straight away

5 Seek advice from your consultant

6 Take a detailed history and fully examine the child for any other injuries

7 Take the child away from mum in A&E and tell her you suspect NAI

8 You cannot be certain that this is NAI so you do nothing, arrange ENT follow up and discharge the child

14.26 You are a foundation year 2 doctor working in the acute assessment unit (AAU). You have clerked an elderly lady and have written up her medications on the drug chart. By mistake you prescribe carbamazepine instead of carbimazole. Later in your shift you review the patient, check the drug chart and notice your mistake. The patient has had one dose and apart from feeling a little dizzy appears fine. What should you do?

Choose the three most appropriate options from the list below.

1 Alert other staff so that she can be monitored for any further symptoms

2 Ask the nurse in charge for advice

3 Consult your defence organisation

4 Delete the medication, not informing other staff or the patient

5 Explain to the patient what has happened, apologise and reassure her that the dizziness will pass and she will not be left with any lasting effects

6 Fill in an incident/significant event report

7 Write a new drug chart and discard the old one

ANSWERS

14.1   1 2 4 3

This question focuses on balancing local evidence-based guidelines, patient choice and the problems faced when dealing with colleagues whose views may differ from our own. It is in the area of professional integrity and backing your own judgement. It is irrelevant whether this man is a real doctor, but having said that, if he is, it will be diplomatically challenging to differ from his opinion being his junior. Asking for his qualifications may just prove difficult and not help matters. We are told to respect patients' ideas, concerns and expectations but not at the expense of practising good medicine. It is always useful to ask a colleague for advice.

14.2   4 2 3 1

This question is about professional integrity, sensitivity to colleagues and concern for patients' welfare. It may be that you can help her with support and advice and if not you, her consultant may be best placed. However, if she is underperforming, we have a duty to 'whistle blow' and management will need informing. Covering for her may overburden you and endanger patient safety.

14.3   3 1 2 4

This is another question about professional integrity and respect for patient confidentiality. Relatives do often ask to speak with doctors about their own concerns. Often these relate to the technical aspects of management, as the terms used can be confusing and worrying for people with no medical background. Allowing them time and space to air their concerns is often enough, and reassures them that you will care for their loved one. If there are any specific questions relating to the patient, or prognosis, you need to be careful not to disclose any confidential information. Gently explaining that you have a duty to keep this information confidential, but are happy to listen to any information they feel would be important for you to know, will often be satisfactory. When a patient indicates they would like you to share certain information with their relatives, it may be appropriate to discuss this with them in the presence of the patient. However, use caution when answering a patient's questions in front of others, as the patient may not know where the answers will lead.

14.4   1 4 3 2

This question is in the area of coping with pressure, finding strategies to cope and not losing sight of the wider picture. Due to recent changes in medical education, there are many more doctors rotating through general practice than ever before and places need to be found for everyone. This means it may be difficult to provide dedicated accommodation for foundation doctors, and the team may not all be familiar with this role. It is important early on to establish with your trainer what your objectives are from this training. Sitting in on surgeries with your trainer and other doctors is an important element, as is learning more about the other members of the primary health care team. However, you will be expected to see patients in your own surgeries, even if occasionally at unusual times. If access to your own surgeries is a consistent problem it may be best to discuss this with the practice manager, who may be able to reorganise other activities in the practice to allow this. The practice manager can let you know when consulting rooms are free when members of staff are away. It is unreasonable to have to put up with this every day so, if no attempt is made to introduce more flexibility, the programme director would need to review the suitability of the practice for training.

14.5   4 3 2 1

This question is in the area of professional integrity and empathy/ sensitivity. The patient may genuinely wish to reward you so it is easy to offend if the gift is quickly rebuffed. However it may be best to explore sensitively for less appropriate motives or if the patient can really afford the gift. It would be inappropriate to accept the gift on one's own behalf. Many practices do have policies (eg buying equipment, patient fund) for dealing with gifts and those over £100 should be registered (Health and Social Care Bill, 2000). Doctors will vary in their reaction to such a gift but as long as the practice policy is not one of outright refusal then the ranking above seems reasonable.

14.6   1 2 3 4

This question is in the area of empathy/sensitivity, responding to the needs of a colleague but also professional integrity, looking at the risks for patients. This question is tricky and there is more than one approach. Depending on your relationship with the colleague, you can speak to them directly, though this may be difficult or intimidating, especially if he is a senior colleague. Discussing it among your other colleagues first helps to encourage ownership of an important issue and aids the gathering of views and information. If you find that your concerns are well founded, your consultant needs to be involved and ultimately the GMC. Alcoholism calls fitness to practise into question. Your colleague should be supported medically although you should not be medically involved in treating him.

14.7   4 2 3 1

This question deals with the concepts of empathy, sensitivity and professional integrity. You made a clinical judgement which has now been questioned – how should you react? A senior colleague has told you that you have omitted a test he would see as essential; it would look negligent to ignore this. You need to consider whether you really did miss a test out and be open to learning from these situations, or you might have been right. It certainly warrants further discussion with the registrar especially if you are confident in your decision. The patient may have some views on this and may have improved or deteriorated depending on her physical pathology or emotional state. She may be reassured or worried by the test, and she may be made more anxious by coming in. It is fair to discuss it with her, but you must do so sensitively, taking into account her ideas, concerns and expectations.

14.8   3 2 4 1

This question raises issues of empathy and sensitivity, and dealing with a potentially stressful situation. We must realise that many processes may have taken place before any encounter between doctor and patient in the consulting room. The patient may have had an unfavourable experience with a member of staff, but we must act in a non-judgemental way and not take sides. It is important to empathise with the patient, and this could just be a way for them to 'let off steam', and they may not wish to take things further. However, in some instances, people may wish to make a formal, written complaint and so they should be aware of the procedure. If the issue is to be raised with the staff member then a senior member of the practice should do so.

14.9   3 2 4 1

This question is in the area of professional integrity. Patient records are confidential and should only be accessed by relevant staff for relevant reasons. There may be a plausible explanation in this case, but if there is not then this needs to be addressed. There may be other aspects of inappropriate behaviour or breaches of privacy in the practice, and this needs to be dealt with from a senior level. Your trainer should be able to provide guidance on how best to deal with this.

14.10   3 4 1 2

This is about coping under pressure as well as empathy/sensitivity. The opinion of other professionals needs to be taken into account – but remember that you have seen the patient more recently and the others are specifically seeking to avoid admission. The patient's views are also important but if admission is really unnecessary clinically, then you should not be persuaded by him. You should be sensitive to this man's home circumstances. If he is agreeable 'rapid response' may be able to provide adequate short-term domiciliary support.

14.11   2 1 3 4

The fear here is that this woman may be storing medication for a suicide attempt. The doctor is under pressure because of this and the time pressures. Some people lead chaotic lives so it is possible the tablets have gone missing or been mislaid. Empathy and sensitivity are important. The doctor should stay calm. It is his/her decision whether to prescribe so a proper assessment of suicide risk can be made and, if it is felt to be low, a prescription can be issued. This is professional integrity and backing one's own judgement. Given the circumstances it is important to liaise with colleagues and issue only a small amount of medication. Doctors can be too trusting, so to issue the full prescription before knowing the whole story may be foolish.

14.12   4 3 1 2

This is a difficult scenario but it is important to address the cause of the bruises, otherwise you could be seen to be colluding with the perpetrator. Addressing this sensitively when the woman is present in the room on her own is important rather than in front of any third party, who could also be involved. If she is not ready to tell you, you must realise that she may be fearful or guilty or anxious, so it is important to build trust so that she can seek help from you when appropriate. You would like to have her permission before involving an outside agency, but this may not always be forthcoming and you will want to act in her best interest as you see it. The question tests empathy and sensitivity responding to and understanding the woman's needs and concerns while at the same time maintaining an appropriate distance and not becoming oversensitive as if personally involved.

14.13   2 1 3 4

This question is about professional integrity. The General Medical Council has recently updated its guidance in *Duties of a Doctor*. Here it states that 'You must not use your professional position to establish or pursue a sexual or improper emotional relationship with a patient or someone close to them'. This is generally taken to mean that relationships with patients or their relatives are considered inappropriate, even if the patient has been discharged from your care, if you met through your professional work. This is partly due to the special nature of the doctor–patient relationship, which means patients or relatives often confide intimate and private thoughts and feelings at times of great stress, and may not feel the same once things settle. In the above situation, the patient's judgement may be impaired by several factors, including the anaesthetic, social isolation, unfamiliar surroundings, frightening clinical procedures and by the pain that they are experiencing. For these reasons he/she may feel attraction to someone in a position of caring. He/she needs to trust that the doctor will not misuse this position. In general as the doctor it is your responsibility to understand the reasons behind the request for a date, and treat the matter sensitively and professionally. However, if you feel intimidated by advances made by a patient, it is a good idea to discuss your feelings with a trusted senior colleague.

14.14   3 4 1 2

In the first instance you should discuss your workload with the consultant, as they will be aware of the sickness absence and may already have considered alternatives. It will be helpful if you can present them with ideas for a solution to the problem. As a junior member of the team you should be supernumerary and not relied on. However, in practice it is difficult for the team to provide sufficient training opportunities on a regular basis without starting to depend on the presence of the junior. It is a good idea to make sure the outpatient department is aware of the situation, as sufficient patients will have been booked to provide you with training, which means that in your absence the clinic is likely to over-run and they need to explain this to patients. Also, it will help them to manage the bookings and cancellations for the next few weeks. If you merely cover the ward for the next few weeks you may miss valuable theatre training opportunities. Personally asking colleagues to cover your bleep would be one option. However, everyone is busy and any contingencies for cover should be ratified by the consultant, as they may have had other plans for reorganising the team during this period.

14.15   4 2 1 3

This question is mainly about planning ahead to ensure that work and family life are compatible. If you are to survive being a successful doctor with young children (at any stage of your career) you need to have contingency plans to cope with this sort of pressure. You may not be able to immediately drop everything to pick up your child from nursery. Colleagues and friends may be able to help and you need to be prepared to ask, and offer help in return. Other systems may not be ideal (such as the ability of a nursery to care for a sick child, or sick leave rules), but you will just have to work around them.

14.16   2 1 3 4

This is an embarrassing situation potentially for doctor and patient but will inevitably happen occasionally. It is not practical to make sure everyone knows where you work. In deciding the best options you need to think about the principles of autonomy, beneficence and non-maleficence. Autonomy usually wins but your patient must not come to harm. Only they will know if seeing a doctor they know in another situation will affect their view of the care received. Obviously you will act professionally and uphold confidentiality and should ensure they are clear about this. You should not treat family or friends as there is a risk of making emotionally involved decisions.

14.17   1 4 3 2

It is important to explore with the patient why she has not told her family about the fact that she is HIV positive and to find out what her worries and concerns are. You need to discuss with her that she is potentially putting her husband and other family members at risk of contracting HIV and find out whether she was aware of this. You should encourage her to tell her husband. You can offer to discuss the issue with her husband whilst she is there but emphasise that it should be her breaking the news and that you are there for support and to answer any questions. Ignoring the issue should be the last resort. This question is in the area of empathy and sensitivity.

14.18   2 3 4 1

DKA is a potentially life threatening condition and needs to be treated as quickly as possible. Explain that if the condition is treated promptly and effectively she should only need to stay in for a few days. You should do everything you can to make sure that the patient does not go home untreated. Showing empathy and sensitivity towards the patient and her problems regarding childcare should help you to formulate a plan with her as how best to solve this problem. The first point of call should be to contact a relative who would be able to pick up the child and care for him while she is in hospital. Failing this you could phone a friend or neighbour that she would be happy for him to stay with. If you are unable to solve the problem this way then you can contact social services as they have a duty to ensure that the boy is cared for.

14.19   1 4 5 3 2

This is a novel situation and unlikely to be encountered in day to day practice but it raises issues regarding efficacy of treatments and what is allowed to be practised within the National Health Service. Certainly in some surgeries, trained acupuncturists see patients and can help in many conditions. Usually, these are musculoskeletal problems. In the hospital setting, there may be several barriers to this type of treatment. It would need to be discussed at a higher level and with relevant advice from the hospital ethics committee and possibly your defence society. The question is about empathy and sensitivity and acting in an open and non-judgemental manner.

14.20   5 1 3 4 2

There is a temptation to do nothing and the short-term placements and frequent changes in rotation often mean that no action is taken in these situations. However, it is likely that the person taking over from you will come under the same stresses and strains caused by the colleague. Finding out from the registrar why he is treating you this way is a good starting point. He may not be aware that he is causing you any distress and you may be able to solve the matter amicably. Your consultant is probably the best point of call if this fails as he/she is in direct working contact with your registrar and may be able to intervene early to improve your working conditions. If you speak to the BMA or the nurses they will probably advise the first two options. Coping with pressure and professional integrity are both issues in this situation.

14.21   2 3 4

As a junior member of the team in a training role, it is assumed that you will have access to senior colleagues for difficult situations such as interpreting X-rays. There is a learning curve for all grades of junior doctor, and the fail-safe mechanism of formal radiology reporting is in place to detect fractures that are subtle and otherwise may be missed. If the patient were to complain in such a case, it would be the responsibility of the consultant to respond, although you may be asked for your input when they are drafting this response. It is also their responsibility to determine the action taken with juniors under these circumstances, and it may be that in this case all the juniors would benefit from additional radiology training. It is clearly wrong to amend patient case notes after the event. Being able to admit mistakes and learn from them is part of professional integrity.

14.22   1 4 5

Working in the Emergency Department is a busy job with the need for 24-hour cover. It is difficult to find locum cover at short notice and doctors are advised to give as much notice as possible of leave requests. However, there will be times when colleagues ask favours at short notice, and there is a need to be flexible, without compromising your ability to function safely. To simply refuse may lead to a difficult working relationship, particularly in the Emergency Department where staff need to pull together as a team. Discussing the matter with your colleague's consultant may make him reassess the importance of this course or the consultant may take steps to provide cover. Allowing your consultant the chance to suggest a solution and offering flexibility in your shifts is one option, but working together as a team to swap shifts and find a solution that suits everyone would also be good. This solution would obviously need ratification and when changing rotas care should be taken to ensure people are clear about when they are expected to be in the department. The question is mainly in the area of empathy and sensitivity, responding to the needs of others with understanding.

14.23   2 3 4

This question tests coping with pressure. This woman is behaving unacceptably but does have a chronic illness and may have problems that you are unable to pick up over the telephone. It would be inappropriate to address her behaviour directly as it may make her worse and risk complaints. It is worth trying to explore why she is behaving like this and not attempting to put her down. However, she needs to be given realistic expectations.

CHAPTER 14 ANSWERS

14.24   1 4 5

This situation needs addressing promptly, and you need to take personal responsibility for this issue, rather than hoping the patient may respond to your letter. With a telephone call you know the patient has received your message. You need to be open and honest about the delay as it may have a bearing on clinical outcome. Non-disclosure is only justified if you think it will adversely affect the patient's mental well-being. Obviously, you should also explain what severe dyskaryosis is. It is important that this incident is looked into further, to ensure it does not happen again. Therefore discussion at a practice significant event meeting openly and honestly is part of the learning from this incident. You may also choose to write to the patient to outline what processes have been remedied to avoid a repeat of the incident (eg designated clinician receiving all smear results and correlating them with a logbook of smears taken to avoid omissions). The question tests professional integrity.

14.25   3 5 6

Taking a detailed history and carrying out a thorough examination are crucial in such cases and enable you to collate all the facts and come to an informed decision about what to do next. It is possible that a perforated eardrum in a child this young could be caused by otitis media and not NAI.

Involving seniors at an early stage is important and given that you are working in the Emergency Department it would seem more appropriate to approach your own consultant before involving the paediatric team. It is more appropriate if your seniors report children to social services. It may be helpful for you to enquire as to whether the child is already on the child protection register in an attempt to obtain more background information on the family.

Taking the child away from mum straight away is likely to increase anxiety and tension surrounding the situation, you need to ensure that the child is safe in the department but there is no need to separate the family straight away. If this is NAI, mum may not be the person responsible for it.

This question involves professional values and highlights the need to trust your clinical judgment and act in the best interests of the child.[1]

14.26   1 5 6

Medications errors are easy to make when you are rushed and managing several tasks at once and particularly if drugs have similar names. It is important to inform both the patient and other staff looking after her so that, if she experiences any other non-specific temporary symptoms that could be accounted for by carbamazepine, the team are aware. The patient should appreciate your honesty and will be grateful for the reassurance about her dizziness. It is important to fill out an incident report at the time of the event. Rewriting the chart and discarding the old one and doing nothing to the drug chart are not appropriate and not in the best interest of the patient. It is better to speak to a more senior doctor rather than a nurse if you need further advice about what to do. There is no need to involve the defence organisation unless the patient makes a complaint. This question is in the areas of coping with pressure and professional values.

REFERENCE

1.   BMA. *Doctors' responsibilities in child protection cases.* (homepage on the Internet), June 2004 (cited 2008 May 10). Available from http://www.bma.org.uk/ap.nsf/content/childprotection

CHAPTER 14 ANSWERS

INDEX

Locators refer to question number.